MANICURE
AND PEDICURE
Handbook

Joy Morris

FSHBTh, IBD, Teacher's Certificate in Further Education

B T Batsford Limited   London

© Joy Morris 1986
First published 1986

Typeset by Servis Filmsetting Ltd, Manchester
and printed in Great Britain by
Anchor Brendon Ltd
Tiptree, Essex
Published by B T Batsford Ltd
4 Fitzhardinge Street, London W1H 0AH

British Library Cataloguing in Publication Data

Morris, Joy
  Manicure and pedicure handbook.
  1. Beauty, Personal   2. Hand—Care and hygiene
  3. Foot—Care and hygiene
  I. Title
  646.7'27   RA776

ISBN 0-7134-4717-6

Contents

Acknowledgment

The author wishes to express very grateful thanks and appreciation for the help and illustrations so kindly provided by the following people: Mr E Harrison and Mr Bernard Simon and staff of Mavala International Ltd; Mrs Renska Mann, Jackie Fisher and Delia Collins of Scholl UK Ltd; Mrs Yani Martin of Fabricius Martin Ltd; Ernest Jackson & Co. Ltd; Neville Morris for his art work; N W Morris for his photographs; Mrs Jane Barton for her preparation and typing of the manuscript, and last but not least, the students of the Bristol College of Electrolysis and Beauty Therapy for creating the need for such a textbook.

Bristol   J M   1986

The product of a professional manicure

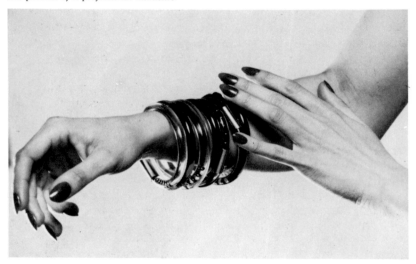

Introduction

The human body is a complex and extremely versatile living machine. As with all machinery it requires servicing and general care to keep it in good functioning order and to make its appearance pleasing to the eye.

The healthy functioning maintenance of the body is the province of specialised medical practitioners such as doctors, dentists, chiropodists and a whole host of allied professions.

The appearance of the body, however, and the resulting effect that appearance has on the morale of the client is the work of the beauty therapist. In order to carry out even the most basic of work on the human body it is necessary for the therapist to have a working knowledge of the way the body is constructed, and its method of functioning.

For those students wishing to study to the accepted level of the major examining authorities the following chapters on anatomy and physiology have been compiled. They are, however, a brief outline of the subject, and students wishing a more 'in depth' study are advised to obtain a specialist book on the subject.

The student who wishes only to acquire the practical skills may pass on to the instructional chapters and illustrations. Students studying alone will be capable of performing the treatments adequately if they follow the routines outlined in the relevant chapters. However, those studying within the supervision of a qualified teacher are recommended to refer to this book as a supplement to their teacher's own class notes.

1 Anatomical structure

Bone structure of the hand, wrist and forearm; Physiology of the hand and forearm; Muscles of the hand, wrist and forearm; Blood circulation with special reference to the hand and foot; Bone structure of the lower leg, ankle and foot; Muscles of the lower leg, ankle and foot; Composition of nail and surrounding tissue

When studying any subject for the first time, the problem arises of terminology appertaining to the subject being new and unfamiliar. This can be confusing and the terminology of anatomy and physiology is no exception to the rule. The following glossary of terms is included for your guidance:

Abduction	Movement away from the centre line of the body
Adduction	Movement towards the centre line of the body
Anterior	Towards the front or the front face of a bone or limb
Aponeurosis	A tendon with a flat sheet-like formation which permits a wider attachment area
Articulation	The movement between two parts of a joint
Articular surface	The area of a bone which meets the articulating surface of another bone. Some of these joints have movement and some do not
Axilla	The underarm cavity or armpit
Cartilage	A strong elastic substance having a variety of uses in the body. One of its principal functions is to act as a buffer between joints and also to prevent jarring between bones when articulation takes place.
Deep	Further away from the surface of the body
Depressor	A muscle which lowers a moving part
Digits	Fingers
Distal	That end of a bone or limb which is farthest away from the body
Dorsal	The upper surface of the feet
Extensor	A muscle which when contracting straightens or extends a joint
Fascia	A sheet of fibrous tissue under the skin
Flexor	A muscle which when contracting brings closer the two parts which it connects. Acts in opposition to an extensor
Inferior	Below, or the lower surface
Inter	Between
Intra	Within
Insertion	A muscle attachment point
Lateral	Towards the outer side
Levator	A muscle which lifts
Ligament	Bands or sheets of fibrous tissue which help support the bones at joints. They are closely

	blended with the periosteum of the bone
Medial	Towards the mid-line of the body
Origin	The attachment point of a muscle, usually the more stationary point, while the Insertion is usually the moveable point
Plane	A flat surface
Plantar	The under surface of the foot
Popliteal	The area behind the knee
Posterior	At the back, or rear view of
Pronation	To rotate the forearm so that the palms are facing down
Proximal	The end of a muscle or bone which is nearest to the body
Rotator	Muscle which turns limbs
Superficial	Nearer to the surface of the body
Superior	The upper surface
Supination	To rotate the forearm so that the palms are upper facing
Sphincter	A muscle which surrounds and closes an orifice or opening such as the eye or mouth
Tendon	A strong band of white fibrous tissue which attaches a muscle to a bone

Approximately 206 bones form the framework or skeleton of the human body to which all the softer structures and organs are attached. The skeleton is both a protection and support to the rest of the body.

Bone is a white fibrous living tissue, ossified (made hard) by the depositing of calcium salts, mainly calcium phospate. It is composed of about one part organic matter and two parts inorganic. Chemical tests have proved that if a piece of bone is soaked in acid, the inorganic matter will dissolve. The bone still retains its shape but becomes soft and pliable. This test proves that the bone owes its hardness, strength and durability to the inorganic content.

The organic content of bone consists of bone cells, blood vessels and marrow. Marrow is a fatty substance which fills the cavities of bones, and its function is the formation of red blood cells.

There are two kinds of bone tissue – cancellous and compact.

The *compact tissue* forms the hard bony substance found in the shaft of long bones and on the outside of flat bones. Minute blood vessels are passed through the compact tissue by a system of small passages called *Haversian canals*.

The *cancellous tissue*, which is more spongelike in appearance, is a framework of bony tunnels through which the blood vessels and nerves pass. This type of tissue is found in the interior of bones, on the ends of bone shafts in long bones, and in very thin bones.

Bones may be classified according to their shape and are usually divided into:

1 *Long bones*, eg tibia, fibula, femur
2 *Short bones*, eg carpal and tarsal bones
3 *Flat bones*, eg bones of the skull, frontal, occipital
4 *Irregular bones*, eg the hip bone or vertebrae. This group includes bones called sesamoid (meaning seed) bones. They are small bones which are developed in tendons. The patella is such a bone and there are other sesamoids found in the tendons of the short muscles of the big toe.

Most *long bones* consist of three main parts – head, shaft and base. The surfaces of the bones which come into contact with or move over other bones are called *articular surfaces*. These are smooth and covered with an articular cartilage. The rest of the bone is covered by a tough fibrous tissue called *periosteum*. Periosteum is a fibrous membrane, the function of which is to provide an attachment for tendons and ligaments and to carry a rich supply of nerves and blood vessels which bring nutrients to the bone. A bone which loses or has its periosteum damaged will die. In addition to the periosteal blood supply, long bones have a special artery which enters the bones and flows into the medullary cavity which is the space within the centre of the bone.

The *short* and *irregular bones* consist almost entirely of cancellous bone of differing degrees of density, surrounded by a thin layer of compact bone. They have no medullary cavity and rely entirely on their periosteal blood supply.

The *flat bones* of the skull contain a thin layer of cancellous bone sandwiched between two layers of thick compact bone.

The circulatory system

In order to live, every organ and tissue of the body needs a regular supply of nutrients. The human blood is a fluid called *plasma* which acts as a carrier of these nutrients, and also performs other necessary functions.

As well as carrying nutrients to the tissues it carries away carbon dioxide and other waste products. The red blood cells carried by the plasma convey oxygen to the tissues and the white blood cells carry most of the protective substances which are able to fight bacteria in the body.

Proteins which are necessary for the building and replacement of tissues are also carried by the plasma, which then carries away the waste products to the organs of excretion.

Enzymes, hormones and other internal secretions are transported from organ to organ by the blood.

The heart is the main organ of the circulatory system which forces the blood around the body via the blood vessels. Arteries are the main routes of transport for blood leaving the heart, these in turn sub-divide into much smaller vessels called *arterioles*. The tissues are bathed in blood from an even smaller network of vessels called *capillaries*. The de-oxygenated blood then filters through a network of collecting capillaries which feed it back into veins. These are the main blood vessels which return the blood to the heart.

Exuding through and bathing all the tissues is a fluid called *lymph*. This fluid collects all the waste products and filters them through collecting points called *lymphatic glands*.

Blood supply of hand and arm

The radial and ulnar arteries are the main suppliers of blood to the hand and arm. They arise from the brachial artery and extend down the inner and outer sides of the arm. The radial artery and its branches supply the thumb side of the arm and the back of the hand. The ulnar artery and its branches supply the little finger side of the arm and palm of the hand.

The main veins returning the blood run almost parallel with the arteries and in most cases take the same name. However, the veins are much more superficial and nearer the surface than the arteries which are buried deeper into the tissues.

Blood supply of leg and foot
The main blood supply to the leg and foot comes from the femoral artery which, when it reaches the area behind the knee becomes the popliteal artery. It then sub-divides into the anterior and posterior tibial arteries.

The two main superficial veins which drain the foot and leg are the short saphenous vein and the long saphenous vein.

It is these two main veins of the leg which often develop an unpleasant condition known as varicose veins.

The leg veins are also accompanied by a series of lymphatic drainage ducts with a set of lymphatic glands in the space behind the knee which is known as the *popliteal* space.

Bones of the arm, wrist and hand

Any study of the human hand will reveal that it is a masterpiece of technical engineering and is a complex structure capable of thousands of intricate movements. It is also capable of performing the most exacting and delicate skills. Apart from a few of the ape species, no other animal has the ability and control over its limbs than has Man.

To appreciate this ability the therapist should be familiar with the intricate arrangement of small bones, joints and muscles which form the hand, wrist and arm and which are detailed next.

Bones of the arm (figure 1)

The *humerus* is the long bone which forms the upper arm, and while it does not concern the therapist involved in performing a manicure, it is essential to know about it as so many of the main muscles of arm movement either attach to or originate from it.

It articulates at its upper end with the scapula to form the rotating joint of the shoulder. The base of the humerus divides into two articular areas called *condyles*.

One of these condyles at the base of the humerus articulates with the upper end of the radius and the other with the second bone of the forearm, which is the ulna.

This joint, which we call the elbow, is a hinge joint which is capable of flexion and extension.

The *radius* and *ulna*, which form the forearm, also articulate with each other and are bound together by a fibrous annular ring;

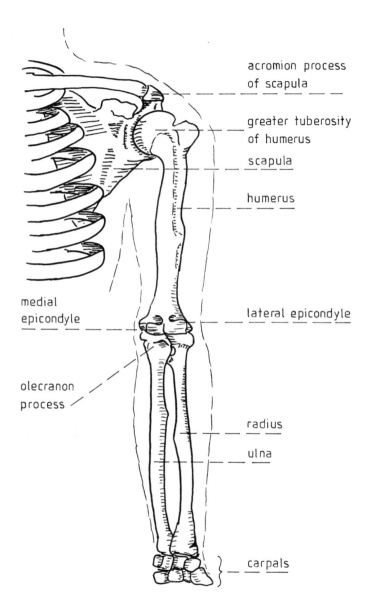

acromion process
of scapula

greater tuberosity
of humerus

scapula

humerus

lateral epicondyle

medial
epicondyle

olecranon
process

radius

ulna

carpals

1 *Bones of the arm*

this binds the two bones together yet allows a rotating movement in which the bones pass over each other. Between these two bones is a tough band of fibrous tissue called the *interosseus membrane*. This protects both bones from impact with each other and also absorbs any shock from a blow to the hand.

The joint between the radius and ulna permits a movement called *pronation*. This is when the radius moves obliquely across the ulna so that the thumb side of the hand is closest to the body. The movement called *supination* takes the thumb side of the hand back to the lateral side.

Bones of the hand and wrist (figure 2)

The bones of the hand are arranged in three groups. They are the *carpals*, the *metacarpals* and the *phalanges*.

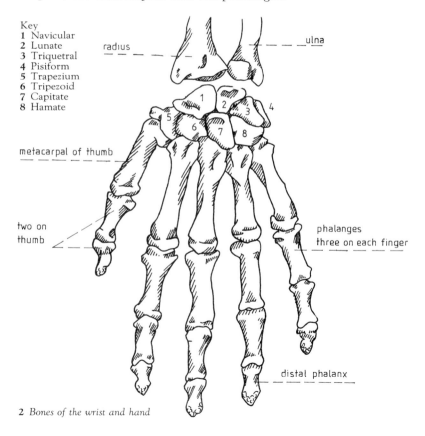

Key
1 Navicular
2 Lunate
3 Triquetral
4 Pisiform
5 Trapezium
6 Tripezoid
7 Capitate
8 Hamate

radius

ulna

metacarpal of thumb

two on thumb

phalanges
three on each finger

distal phalanx

2 *Bones of the wrist and hand*

The carpus
This is a flexible joint which we call the wrist and is made up of eight carpal bones which are cuboidal in shape. Their sides have articulating surfaces where they make joints with each other, and they are arranged in two rows, with four bones to a row. They are all held by ligaments which bind them together.

Starting on the thumb side the upper row are:

1   Navicular (scaphoid)
2   Lunate (semilunar)
3   Triquetral (cunieform)
4   Pisiform
    The lower row also starting on the thumb side:
5   Trapezium
6   Trapezoid
7   Capitate
8   Hamate

The joint where the carpal bones articulate with the radius permits four types of movement which give much of the deftness associated with the use of the hand. They are:

1   Flexion
2   Extension
3   Abduction
4   Adduction

By using these movements in a sequence pattern the hand can perform a complete circular movement.

The metacarpals
These five long slim bones make up the palm of the hand, and are numbered one to five. Their bases articulate with the appropriate carpal bones and their heads with the bones of the fingers. The metacarpals are joined together by interosseus muscles which are attached to the shafts of the bones.

The phalanges or digits
The fingers of the hands are comprised of a series of small long bones arranged end to end. There are three bones to each finger but only two to the thumb.

The fleshy pad on the palm side of the hand, which lies over the first metacarpo-phalangeal joint at the base of the thumb is known as the *thenar eminence*, and the similar pad which lies from the fifth metacarpo-phalangeal joint to the wrist (on the small finger side of the palm) is called the *hypothenar eminence*.

Bones of the thigh and leg (figure 3)

The femur
The pedicurist should not concern herself with a detailed study of the femur but should learn its general appearance and shape, and also appreciate that the attachments of many of the calf muscles arise from the distal extremity of this bone. The femur consists of a rounded proximal head which fits into a cup-shaped socket on the hip bone forming the hip joint. The femur then has a strong shaft which is the main body of the thigh and a base which articulates with the patella and head of the tibia thus forming the knee joint.

The patella
The patella is a sesamoid bone developed in the tendon of the extensor muscles of the thigh. It lies to the front of the knee joint of which it forms a part. This tendon is continued distally as the ligamentum patellae, which inserts into the tubercle of the tibia.

The tibia
The tibia or shin bone is the larger of the two long bones in the lower leg and lies on the medial side of the fibula. It articulates proximally with the femur in the formation of the knee joint and with the upper end of the fibula. Distally it articulates with the lower end of the fibula and with the talus to form the ankle joint.

Six of the main muscles of the leg form an attachment to the tibia and they are:

1 Popliteus   (insertion)
2 Soleus   (origin)
3 Tibialis posterior   (origin)
4 Tibialis anterior   (origin)
5 Flexor digitorum longus   (origin)
6 Extensor digitorum longus   (origin)

The Fibula
The fibula is a long narrow bone situated on the lateral side of the

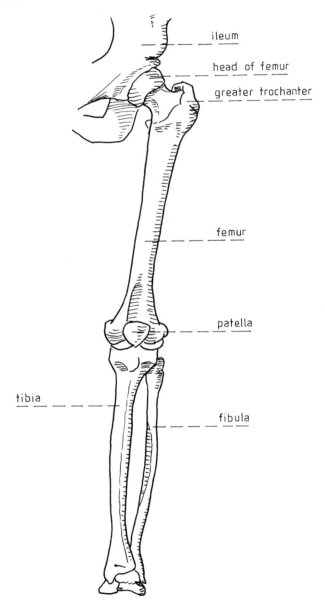

ileum

head of femur

greater trochanter

femur

patella

tibia

fibula

3 *Bones of the thigh and leg*

tibia, with which it articulates at both ends. The ends of the bone are slightly modified and enlarged to form the head proximally and the lateral malleolus distally.

The head articulates with the inferior surface of the lateral condyle of the tibia. Its posterior surface is rough for the attachment of the soleus muscle, which arises from the head and proximal third of the posterior surface of the shaft of the fibula. Anteriorly the head gives origin to the proximal end of the peroneus longus muscle. The distal end of the fibula is called the *lateral malleolus* and forms the lateral bony projection of the ankle joint.

There are eight muscles which attached to the fibula. They are:

1 Flexor hallucis longus   (origin)
2 Tibialis posterior   (origin)
3 Soleus   (origin)
4 Extensor digitorum longus   (origin)
5 Peroneus tertius   (origin)
6 Peroneus longus   (origin)
7 Peroneus brevis   (origin)
8 Extensor hallucis longus   (origin)

Bones of the foot (figures 4 and 5)

The bones of the foot are grouped under the following headings:

The tarsus consisting of:
Talus
Calcaneum
Navicular
Medial, intermediate and lateral cuneiform bones
Cuboid

The metatarsus consisting of:
The five metatarsal bones, numbered one to five from the medial to the lateral side

The phalanges consisting of:
Two for the big toe and three for all the other toes

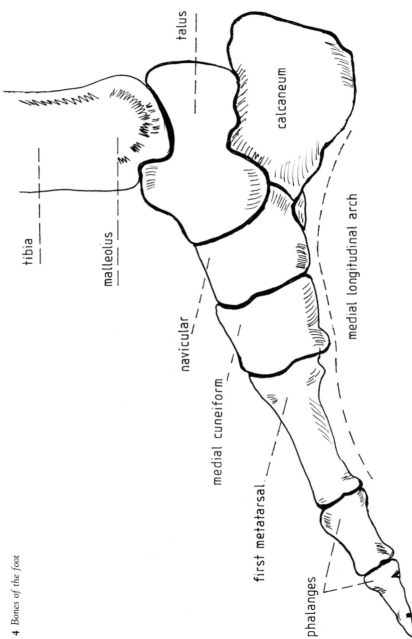

talus

tibia

malleolus

calcaneum

navicular

medial cuneiform

medial longitudinal arch

first metatarsal

phalanges

4 *Bones of the foot*

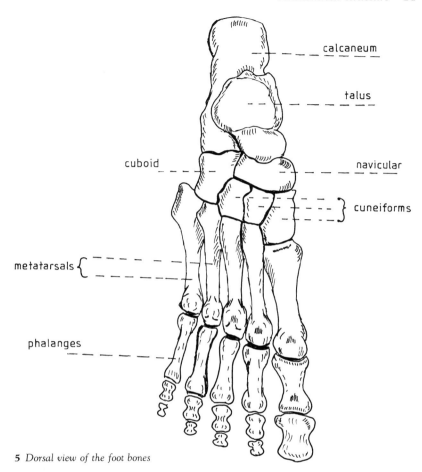

5 *Dorsal view of the foot bones*

The tarsus

The talus
The talus forms the keystone of the arch of the foot and through it the weight of the body is transmitted to the foot. The talus also plays an important part in the formation of the ankle joint.

The calcaneum
The calcaneum is the largest bone in the foot. It supports the talus and articulates with the cuboid anteriorly. The posterior half of

this bone forms the posterior column of the longitudinal arch of the foot and its posterior extremity forms the bony projection of the heel.

Seven muscles attach to the calcaneum. These are:

1   Extensor digitorum brevis   (origin)
2   Flexor digitorum brevis   (origin)
3   Abductor hallucis   (origin)
4   Abductor digiti minimi   (origin)
5   Flexor digitorum accessorius   (origin)
6   Tibialis posterior   (insertion)
7   Tendo Achillis   (insertion)

The navicular
The navicular lies on the medial side of the foot between the talus posteriorly and the three cuneiforms anteriorly.

The muscle attached to the navicular is:

Tibialia posterior   (insertion)

The cuneiform bones
The cuneiform bones lie between the navicular posteriorly and the bases of the first three metatarsal bones anteriorly. They are roughly wedge-shaped and are called medial, intermediate and lateral, according to their position.

The shape and position of the three cuneiforms contribute to the transverse arch of the foot.

The cuboid
The cuboid lies on the lateral side of the foot between the calcaneum posteriorly and the bases of the fourth and fifth metatarsals anteriorly.

Two muscles attach to the cuboid. These are:

1   Flexor hallucis brevis   (origin)
2   Tibialis posterior   (insertion)

The metatarsus
There are five metatarsal bones numbered from the medial to the lateral side. They are classified as long bones and articulate at the head with the phalanges and the bases articulate mainly with the cuneiforms.

The phalanges
The phalanges of the toes are much smaller than the phalanges of the fingers. The big toe has two phalanges but the other toes contain three, although in many cases in the smaller toes the three are very small and ankylosed and appear as one bone.

Arches of the foot

The feet, because they support the entire weight of the body, must be strong and yet, because of the need for comfortable movement, must be flexible. With these two objects in mind, one can see that the foot has evolved into a two-intersecting arch system.

Elasticity is possible because these arches are not rigid structures, but are formed by a series of bones held together by strong but pliable and elastic ligaments and muscles.

The longitudinal arch is the main arch which runs from back to front of the foot with a medial or internal aspect and a lateral aspect. The medial aspect of the longitudinal arch is formed by the calcaneum, the cuboid bone and the two outer metatarsal bones.

The transverse arch has two aspects, a posterior and an anterior. The anterior transverse arch occurs at the level of the heads of the metatarsal bones and flattens out when walking, but returns to shape when the weight is taken off it.

The posterior transverse arch occurs at the tarsal-metatarsal joint and is the most visual part of the transverse arch of the foot.

The muscular system

The muscular system of the body is the system concerned with movement. Every movement made, either voluntarily or involuntarily by or within the body is made by groups of muscles contracting or relaxing. There are over 500 such muscles and they contribute about 40 per cent of the total body weight.

Muscle tissue can only contract or relax and there are several classifications of differing types of muscles, but for the purposes of this book only the striped or voluntary muscles are described.

These voluntary muscles form the rounded contours of the body and are under the control of the will of the individual. Muscles form their attachments to bones, ligaments, tendons and cartilages and in some instances to other muscles.

Each muscle has two attachments, called an *origin* and an

insertion. The origin is usually defined as being attached to the less movable, more fixed or stable bone or attachment. The insertion is fixed to the more movable bone or attachment. The muscle contracts by pulling its insertion back towards the origin. Often a muscle has an origin or insertion into more than one bone or attachment.

Muscles in action always contract or shorten and normally work in pairs, so that when one muscle is contracting and shortening (known as the synergist) another muscle will be relaxing in a checking or steadying movement (known as the antagonist).

Muscles are also classified according to the type of action they perform. These classes are:

Extensors	Extend the limb
Flexors	Flex the limb
Adductors	Move the limb towards the mid-line of the body
Abductors	Take the limb away from the mid-line
Rotators	Rotate the limb
Supinators	Turn the limb upwards
Pronators	Turn the limb downwards
Sphincters	Encircle an opening (such as the mouth)
Eversions	Raise the lateral border of the foot and turn the sole outwards
Inversions	Raise the medial border of the foot and turn the sole inwards

For the purposes of the study of manicure and pedicure it is only necessary to study the most superficial muscles and their effect on the actions of the limbs, so only these have been listed. However, anyone wishing to study the muscular system more fully is recommended to obtain one of the many good books on anatomy and physiology which cover the subject and are readily available.

Muscles of the arm and hand (figures 6 and 7)

The main muscles of the upper arm are:

The deltoid	Origin	The clavicle and scapula
	Insertion	The deltoid tubercle of the humerus

	Action	Abduction of the arm to a right angle from the shoulder
The biceps	Origin	By two tendons from the scapula
	Insertion	Into the radial tuberosity of the radius
	Action	Flexes shoulder and elbow, aids supination of the hand
The triceps	Origin	By three tendons from the scapula and humerus
	Insertion	Into the olecranon process of the ulna
	Action	Extension of the shoulder and elbow

Superficial muscles of the forearm and wrist (figures 6 and 7)

Flexor group

Flexor carpi radialis	Origin	Medial epicondyle of the humerus
	Insertion	Base of the second metacarpal
	Action	Flexes the wrist and adducts the hand
Flexor digitorum sublimis	Origin	The medial epicondyle and the anterior surface of the radius
	Insertion	The middle phalanges of the fingers
	Action	Flexes fingers and wrist
Flexor pollicus longus	Origin	Anterior surface of the radius
	Insertion	Distal phalanx of the thumb
	Action	Flexes the thumb
Brachioradialis	Origin	Lateral side of the humerus
	Insertion	Lower end of the radius above the styloid process
	Action	Flexes the elbow and is often called the 'carrying muscle'

Extensor group

| *Extensor carpi radialis brevis* | Origin | Lateral epicondyle of humerus |

Extensor carpi radialis brevis	*continued*	
	Insertion	Base of third metacarpal
	Action	Extension of wrist and elbow
Extensor carpi ulnaris	Origin	Humerus
	Insertion	Base of fifth metacarpal
	Action	Extends and stabilises the wrist when the hand is clenched
Extensor digitorum	Origin	Humerus
	Insertion	By division into four tendons which insert into the four fingers
	Action	These are the four tendons which can be seen clearly on the back of

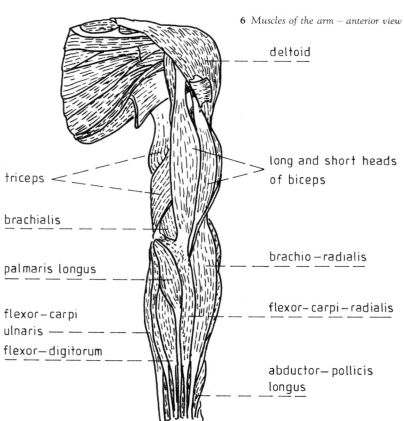

6 *Muscles of the arm — anterior view*

deltoid

long and short heads of biceps

triceps

brachialis

brachio–radialis

palmaris longus

flexor–carpi ulnaris

flexor–carpi–radialis

flexor–digitorum

abductor– pollicis longus

continued

the hand when the hand is extended. They extend the fingers

Extensor pollicus longus	Origin	The shaft of the ulna and the interosseus membrane
	Insertion	The base of the distal phalanx
	Action	Extends the thumb

Rotation muscles

Pronator terres	Origin	The humerus
	Insertion	Into the shaft of the radius
	Action	It rotates the radius to turn the palm of the hand backwards

7 *Muscles of the arm – posterior view*

deltoid

triceps

triceps tendon

terris major

olecranon

anconeus

flexor carpi —
ulnaris

extensor carpi—
ulnaris

extensor digitorum

Muscles of the lower leg (figure 8)

Tibialis anterior   Origin   Tibia

Insertion   By means of a tendon into the
medial cuneiform and the base of
the first metatarsal bone

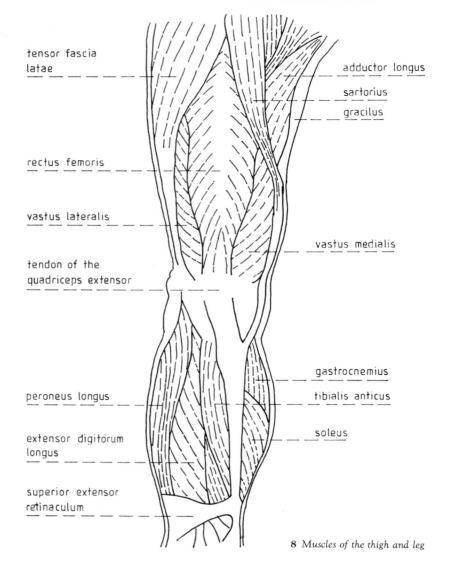

tensor fascia
latae

adductor longus

sartorius

gracilus

rectus femoris

vastus lateralis

vastus medialis

tendon of the
quadriceps extensor

gastrocnemius

peroneus longus

tibialis anticus

extensor digitórum
longus

soleus

superior extensor
retinaculum

8 *Muscles of the thigh and leg*

	Action	Flexes the ankle, inverts and adducts the foot
Extensor hallucis longus	Origin	Fibula
	Insertion	By means of a tendon into the base of the distal phalanx of the big toe
	Action	Extends big toe and flexes ankle
Extensor digitorum longus	Origin	Tibia and fibula
	Insertion	By means of four tendons into the four lateral toes
	Action	Flexes the ankle and extends the four lateral toes
Peroneus longus	Origin	Fibula
	Insertion	The lateral malleolus, calcaneum, cuboid, medial cuneiform and base of first metatarsal bone
	Action	Extends ankle, everts the foot and helps to maintain both longitudinal and transverse arch
Peroneus brevis	Origin	Fibula
	Insertion	Calcaneum and base of the fifth metatarsal bone
	Action	Extends ankle and everts the foot
Gastrocnemius	Origin	By two heads from the medial and lateral epicondyles of the femur
	Insertion	The two fleshly bodies of this muscle join into a broad membranous tendon and blend with that of the soleus and sometimes the plantaris to form the Achilles tendon. This attaches to the posterior surface of the calcaneum
	Action	Flexes the knee and extends the ankle
Plantaris	Origin	Femur
	Insertion	Achilles tendon and calcaneum
	Action	Aids in the flexing of the knee and extension of the ankle

Soleus	Origin	Tibia and fibula
	Insertion	By means of the Achilles tendon into the posterior surface of the calcaneum
	Action	Extensor of the ankle
Popliteus	Origin	Femur
	Insertion	Tibia
	Action	Flexes and medially rotates the knee
Tibialis posterior	Origin	Tibia and fibula
	Insertion	Medial malleolus, navicular and tarsal and some metatarsals
	Action	Extends the ankle and inverts the foot, but also plays an important part in maintaining the arch of the foot
Flexor digitorum longus	Origin	Tibia
	Insertion	Bases of distal phalanges
	Action	Extends and inverts the foot, but also plays an important part in maintaining the arch of the foot
Flexor hallucis longus	Origin	Fibula
	Insertion	Tibia and talus and base of distal phalanx
	Action	Extends the ankle and flexes the big toe. Also plays an important part in strengthening the arch of the foot

Muscles of the foot

The dorsal aspect of the foot has only one short muscle. That is:

Extensor digitorum brevis	Origin	Calcaneum
	Insertion	Four fleshy bellies which insert by means of tendons into the four medial toes
	Action	Extends the four medial toes, and assists in the adduction of the big toe

The plantar surface or sole of the foot has four layers of muscles. These are all covered superficially by a strong fibrous fascia called the *plantar aponeurosis*.

These are the superficial muscles and their actions which show quite clearly how the muscles are designed to work in groups and also in pairs with an antagonist and a protagonist.

There are of course many more deeper seated muscles as well as a collection of smaller interosseus muscles which work to make the millions of movements possible by the wrist, hand and fingers, the ankle, foot and toes.

Composition of nails (figure 9)

The nails of the human body are translucent plates which cover the upper surfaces of the distal end of the fingers and toes. On a healthy body the nails should be an even, pink colour with a smooth, slightly glossy surface. Although their principal function is that of protection, research has shown that manual dexterity is greatly impaired where the nail is missing.

Tests on people who have either lost their finger nails or were born without them, have shown that they are not so capable of performing the more delicate or dextrous movements such as picking up very small objects or threading needles.

The loss of toenails can also cause some people to experience difficulty in balancing and walking until they have adjusted to the loss.

Continuously growing throughout life, the nails are not shed as the human hair is, but can be badly damaged or in some instances lost by knocks or blows, disease or drug therapy. However, a damaged nail will grow again if the matrix and nail bed are not damaged.

The semi-translucent *nail plate* is composed of layers of keratinised cells, packed very closely together with a fat content but very little moisture. These layers of nail tissue can be seen clearly when the nails have been subjected to a strong external drying agent which has caused the fat and moisture content to dry out. The nails become dry and brittle and separate very clearly into layers. Housewives who continuously immerse their hands in water and strong detergents or bleaching agents often have such nails.

The nail plate is set into a depression or *nail bed* at the distal end of the dorsal or upper surface of the last phalanx of finger or toe.

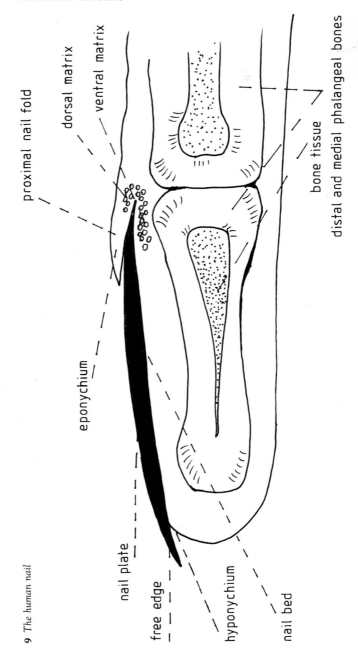

9 *The human nail*

Roughly rectangular in shape, the nail plate has a free edge at its terminal end and at the opposite, proximal end, it inserts under an outgrowth of epidermal cells called the *eponychium* or *cuticle*. The underside of this hard nail plate is grooved by longitudinal ridges and furrows. The nail bed on which it rests has a similar corresponding pattern of grooves and furrows which interlock to form a method of retention.

The nail is not flat, but is normally curved on two planes, transversely and longitudinally. The depth of curve varies with each individual and can sometimes be distorted by occupational pressures. In some pathological conditions the nail can be abnormally curved or flattened and may sometimes appear spoon-shaped.

The nail bed on which the nail plate lies is a thickened layer of epidermis which does not appear to have either a stratum lucidum or granulosum and is without follicles and sweet glands. It does, however, contain a large quantity of prickle cells.

At the proximal end of the nail in the area which is under the eponychium is the *matrix* or growing area of the nail. This matrix also extends around the proximal end of the nail, forming a dorsal and ventral matrix.

Changes in the epidermal cells of this matrix, similar to the keratinisation of those in the superficial epidermis, take place, thus forming the hardened tissue of the nail plate.

A small half-moon shaped area between the matrix and the main body of the nail plate is called the *lunula*. This half-moon shape is clearly visible on most nails near the base of the nail. One theory for its distinctive light appearance is that it is an area where the keratinisation or hardening process of the cells is not complete and because of this the tissue is lighter and the connective tissue looser.

The nail bed and matrix have a rich capillary network arising from the digital arterial arches which are below the nail bed supplying blood by a capillary loop system. There are also many free sensory nerve endings present giving the whole area a greater sensitivity as anyone who has suffered damage to the nail bed can confirm.

The human nail continues to grow all through life and many research projects have studied this rate of growth. Some have put forward the theory that there is a specific growth rate, often quoted as being about 3mm (⅛in.) per month. This can of course be used as a general guide, but as with all human tissue growth and replacement, so many variations occur due to internal and external conditions. One research project claimed that there is a more active growth rate in the summer than winter. This could be true, but may also be due to a change of diet in winter with a lower consumption of certain vitamins and minerals which are contained in the fresh vegetables and fruits of a summer diet.

Age certainly plays a part in the nail growth rate. The nails of children have been shown to grow faster than those of the mature adult, with a positive slowing down of the growth rate in the very elderly.

The growth of the nail is most noticeable where the free edge at the distal end of the nail extends out over the area of tissue known as the *hyponychium*.

The cuticle is a frame of epidermal tissue which grows around the perimeter of the nail plate thus helping to hold it in place. It also functions as a seal to stop infections penetrating to the cells of the nail matrix. The cuticle should be kept soft and supple and not allowed to adhere to the nail plate as it is being extended by growth, otherwise it will be drawn forward, stretched and eventually split causing agnails or 'hang nails'.

2 Tools and materials

Tools and materials used for manicuring and pedicuring including selection, care, correct handling and sterilisation; Preparation
of manicure tray for use

Selection and care of manicure and pedicure equipment

The small tools or instruments necessary to carry out the work of manicure and pedicure should be chosen with great care. Obviously you should purchase the best you can possibly afford, but this does not necessarily mean the most expensive. As with many other aspects of beauty therapy, manicure has seen the coming of very expensive 'gimmicky' tools that have sent some rushing to buy them, only to be left with expensive white elephants that are either difficult or fiddly to use, or just do not stand up to the strain of repeated daily use.

The best place to see a full range of small equipment displayed and to be able to compare quality and prices is at the several professional organisations exhibitions. There the leading stockists display a full range of items and their staff are usually very willing to explain and discuss the merits of the various items. At most exhibitions these days it is possible to purchase there and then, which is much more sensible than sending for something from a catalogue. Obviously items that have a fine ground cutting edge to them are much more expensive, so great care should be taken in your choice.

Heavy duty nail clippers
Usually made of fine Sheffield steel with a ground cutting edge, the heavy duty nail clippers come in a variety of sizes and weights. It is very important to choose a pair which suits your hand size and which does not appear too heavy. When doing an occasional pedicure this would not seem very necessary, but if you spend all day using a pair of nail clippers that are both too heavy to hold and also too difficult to clip with, you will soon see the sense in buying wisely. These can also be purchased with a plastic shield designed to prevent particles of nail from flying into the pedicurist's face and eyes. In repeated use, however, these have been known to come loose and foul the cutting blades. Then they tend to get removed and left off altogether. All nail clippers require sharpening from time to time so it is a good idea to find out from the suppliers if they have a follow-up sharpening service.

When purchasing heavy duty nail clippers or cuticle clippers, you usually find a metal 'spring' inside the handle. This is sometimes in the reverse position, obviously for easy storage, and on purchase should be moved into a position so that there is 'springiness' to the handles. If in doubt ask the supplier to demonstrate it.

Many pedicurists are tending to use the mechanical type clipper manufactured by the Scholl Manufacturing Company. These can be purchased with a plastic outer casing which catches all the cut nail droppings. These are cheap enough to be replaced when blunt, but some maintain that they do not look very professional, although they are very efficient if used correctly.

Cuticle nipper or clipper
These are a much smaller version of the big clippers, but have their finely ground cutting blades at a different angle. The alternative to these nippers is the fine cuticle paring 'knife' manufactured by Revlon.

Cuticle knife
You should look for a fine ground flat blade knife which can be resharpened. So many manicurists work with blunt instruments and then wonder why their work is not as good as it could be. On the other hand you should take care not to have these cuticle knives as sharp as scapels or a great deal of damage could result.

Diamond impregnated file or metal file
These files are only suitable for pedicure work as even the finest grade would be too coarse for manicure. A longer version is much better than a shorter one.

Emery boards
The finest emery boards are those that are reasonably long with a coarse grade one side and a finer grade the other. Some boards are very stiff and most manicurists find that they prefer the thinner, more flexible boards. Cost, however, plays an important part in the selection of emery boards, as it is necessary for hygienic purposes to use a new board on every client.

Rubber hoof stick
Many different types of implements are on the stands intended for the purpose of pushing back the cuticles. Safest by far is either an orange stick wrapped in cotton wool or the rubber hoof stick. These little rubber wedges usually come attached to the end of a shaped wooden implement. As the rubber tends to perish with

repeated sterilisation it is a good practice to buy several at a time and buy them as cheaply as possible.

Orange sticks
These items are much more useful to the manicurist than the manufactured 'cotton bud' because the stems of the orange sticks are not so pliable and 'bendy'. These should be bought in bulk in order to buy as cheaply as possible, because these also should be used only on one client and disposed of at the end of the manicure or pedicure.

Nail buffer
The nail buffer at one time was a standard piece of any manicure box or case, but with the advent of nail varnishes, etc, it lost its popularity. With the increase in male manicure and a leaning of some women towards a much more natural look, nail buffing has become popular again.

A good nail buffer should be large enough to sit comfortably in the hand. They are usually covered in chamois leather but the professional manicurist must obtain one which has the facilities for a disposable cover to be placed over it. Obviously to have a series of chamois leather covers, and wash and sterilise them after each treatment is not practical. Therefore it is advised that a small piece of thin disposable cotton, such as the type of cotton one can sometimes find in strips being used for leg waxing, be adapted and used over the leather, and disposed of after each client.

Hand bowl or manicure dish
A small bowl or dish, large enough to accommodate the clients' fingers and knuckles is sufficient, but the dishes specially manufactured for the purpose look so much more professional. Using them also makes such good sense when you realise that it is practically impossible for the client to spill the water either over herself or the salon carpet!

Electrically heated manicure dish
You can also obtain an electrically heated dish into which oil is poured for a hot oil manicure. As with most electrical equipment you should ensure that it complies to the British Safety Institute Standards and also that you have an electrical wall socket in the vicinity of the manicure chair!

Miscellaneous

Towels and **gowns** should all be readily washable and the surface on which the manicure takes place should also be covered with disposable tissues. Ordinary tissues are obviously too small, but a piece taken from a salon bed roll covers the surface adequately.

Pretty coloured towels to match the décor of the salon or manicure cubicle add a touch of luxury, as does an attractive matching ceramic dish into which the client places her jewellery. Initially these things cost just a little extra, but certainly give the client the impression of luxury as well as hygiene.

The theme of luxury should also be conveyed as much as possible with the selection of the larger items needed to complete the manicure/pedicure area or cubicle. Often you have to utilise the furniture that is available in general use in the salon, such as the main beauty chair. It may also be necessary to limit yourself because of a small amount of space available. However, if space and finance allow, there is now a huge variety of custom-built **manicure tables** and **stools** to be seen at the showrooms. Pretty is not always practical, so it is advisable for the manicurist herself to be present at the purchasing of such equipment so that she can actually try it out for size, manoeuverability and general adaptability. Stools which have storage drawers for towels, etc, and table tops which swivel to allow the client to get in and out of her seat comfortably are all points to be considered.

The ultimate in pedicure cubicle furniture is the ready plumbed-in **foot basin** with running hot and cold water. Of course this has to be accompanied by a chair with a swivel and hydraulic pump action, which most beauty chairs have.

Electric drills are also available from the chiropodial supply houses. They can be obtained with a built-in vacuum suction unit to suck up dust and debris. Pedicurists doing a lot of thick nail shaping and reducing would be advised to consider such a useful item, but they are of course rather expensive.

Some of the manicure supply houses also produce a **custom-built tray** of all their products for the professional manicurist-pedicurist. These usually contain all that is necessary, including a full range of coloured varnishes. These can be supported by also stocking retail sizes for clients to purchase.

Hygiene and sterilisation

It is essential for the manicurist and pedicurist to be aware that infections can be spread from one client to another and serious illnesses could be caused by a seemingly trivial touching of an open or torn cuticle with an unsterile instrument such as a cuticle knife. It is also necessary to know the correct way to avoid any risk of transmitting or infecting anyone in our daily work, or indeed in picking up infections ourselves.

Bacteria are invisible one-celled micro-organisms found everywhere and on everything. They cannot be seen with the naked eye, but a microscope will reveal that they are existing everywhere. They are much more numerous in dirt, decaying animal or vegetable matter and diseased tissue.

There are two main types:

1 *Non-pathogenic*
   These are the harmless type of bacteria which are necessary for normal biological processes to take place.
2 *Pathogenic*
   Commonly known as *germs*, these are responsible for all diseases. This pathogenic group then sub-divides into a series of six different types of bacteria, the names of which need not concern the therapist at this stage.

These germs multiply and grow when conditions are most favourable to them, that is, in warm moist dark damp dirty places. They are then easily transmitted from place to place, usually by human beings. It is necessary that everyone should be aware of this and reduce the unnecessary spread of infections by taking very simple everyday precautions.

It should be a golden rule that no eating matter of any description is brought into the treatment rooms. All staff should wash their hands thoroughly after using the toilet and also before and after touching a client.

The salon and treatment areas should be cleaned thoroughly and regularly, with all surfaces and walls being of materials which can be washed down with an antiseptic solution.

All towels, etc, should be boil-washed and where possible every item should be of a disposable type.

Items such as emery boards and orange sticks should be disposed of immediately to prevent the risk of cross-infection.

There are very many types and methods of sterilisation available, but many of them are too impractical for the average beauty salon or manicure/pedicure cubicle. The safest, most compact method of sterilisation open to the manicurist/pedicurist is the **ultra violet steriliser**. Bacteria cannot live any longer than a few hours when exposed to ultra violet irradiation. The UV sterilisers are now available at most wholesale beauty equipment houses at a reasonable cost. One word of caution, however, when purchasing such a steriliser: check that the door of this type of steriliser has a leak-proof guard as a constant beam of UV light 'leaking' from the steriliser door could prove harmful to an operator sitting constantly in the vicinity of it.

When using the ultra violet light steriliser, bear in mind that light travels in straight lines and unless the light actually strikes the instruments, they cannot become sterile. Care must be taken firstly to wash all instruments in running hot water, brushing with a small nail brush if any debris remains, then place in the steriliser and lay flat so that the light can strike all surfaces. Often, where a steriliser is shared with others, you see instruments being washed, wrapped in a bundle in a tissue then being placed in the steriliser. This is totally useless because the light does not strike the surface of the instruments and they are therefore not sterile.

The therapist must also be aware that sterilisation is not instant. Instruments would need to be in the steriliser for a minimum of one hour or according to the manufacturer's instructions for using the steriliser. It makes good sense in this case to have two or three of every item needed so that you always have them available in a sterile condition and ready for use.

As well as such a steriliser it is important for the therapist to use certain chemicals in an effort to check the spreading of germs. Two types of chemicals are available. These are:

1   *Antiseptics*
    These are ready prepared solutions which may prevent the growth of bacteria without actually killing them. An antiseptic can safely be used on the skin. *Dettol* would be an example of a good antiseptic solution.
        Small instruments should be placed in such a solution on the manicure/pedicure table after removal from the steriliser.
2   *Disinfectants*
    These are usually classed as chemicals which kill germs. There

are a great number of them on the market under proprietory brand names ranging from the phenol groups such as *Lysol* or *Jeyes Fluid*, to much more modern compounds such as *Phisohex* or *Hibitane*.

The student manicurist/pedicurist sometimes gets a little worried by all this talk about bacteria and disease, but if you establish a good efficient routine of hygiene and sterilisation and stick to it religiously then there is little chance of anything going wrong.

But while on the subject of hygiene, it should be said that it is very bad practice for a therapist with a heavy cold or bad cough to continue to see clients. The old war-time adage 'Coughs and sneezes spread diseases' is certainly true when you are in the warm, dry atmosphere of a small salon or treatment cubicle. If it is absolutely imperative that you continue to work, then obtain a pack of disposable face masks from the chemist and keep your germs to yourself.

Contra-indications to manicure
Cuts, bruises or abrasions
Broken bones, swellings or sprains
Skin infections
Fungal infections
Paronychia
Shedding nails
Ingrowing nails
Severely damaged or thin nails
See also chapter 5

---

3 Manicure techniques

Manicuring techniques: filing, cuticle care, nippering, buffing, enamelling and patching; Manicure routine; Hand and forearm massage; Repairing nails, applying false nails

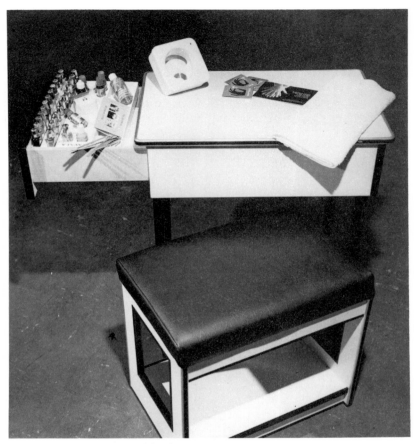

10 *The Mavala manicure stool has been specially designed for salon use. Their professional manicure tray fits neatly into a drawer which can be closed at the end of the day. The stool slides under the table for a tidy appearance*

Materials required for manicure trolley (figure 10)

Manicure trolley, table or tray

Towels and disposable tissues

Small dish containing antiseptic such as *Savlon* or *Dettol* for small instruments to rest in

Manicure cushion (usually a square of foam rubber covered in a removable towelling cover)

Nail clippers or scissors

Emery boards (for hygiene purposes, always a new one for each client)

Cuticle knife

Cuticle nippers

Orange stick

Nail brush

Nail buffer

Paste polish or powder for buffing

Waste container

Cotton wool in hygienic container

Cotton buds

Liquid soap or manicure 'pill'

Cuticle softening oil or cream

Cuticle removing lotion

Massage cream (spatula to remove cream from jar)

Nail varnish remover

A selection of nail enamels both dark and light, frosted and plain

A base protective coat

Top gloss coat

Attractive glass or ceramic dish for client's jewellery

Nail repair and fixative kit

Quick drying spray aerosol

Dilute solution of hydrogen peroxide or proprietory brand of nail stain remover such as *Perox Chlor*

Manicure routine

In order that the client can enjoy her manicure treatment, it is essential that a great deal of care be taken to ensure that she is seated comfortably to begin with and also that the therapist has everything that will be needed to hand. Nothing is more irritating to the client than the therapist who has to leave the treatment area to fetch things.

It is therefore a good idea to have a trolley always set and prepared ready for a manicure, except for the small instruments which should be in the steriliser. It can be the job of a junior member of staff to check that the trolley is always neat and tidy and ready for use, with disposable items always being replenished as required. All pots of colours should be checked to ensure that they have not thickened and become unusable. A good selection of colours should also be stocked with a back-up supply of retail sizes being available as many clients like to purchase the same colour.

It is not good salon policy to pressurise the client into buying retail lines, but it makes good business sense to have a reliable range of nail treatment products and colours available if the clients ask for them.

To commence the manicure treatment, the therapist must ask the client to remove her hand and arm jewellery. A decent-sized elegant and decorative glass or ceramic container should be offered to the client, and the therapist should ask the client to place her rings, watch and bracelets into it. *At no time should this container be placed anywhere other than on the top of the trolley in the client's full view at all times.* This way the salon will not be at risk as far as the loss or mislaying of valuable items are concerned. If the therapist does not handle the jewellery then she cannot be accused of having dropped or damaged it in any way. This may sound petty, but it makes sound business practice for insurance purposes.

Cover the client's clothing with a clean towel or a disposable cover and roll up her sleeves to above the elbow.

A clean tissue should be tucked around the lower edge of the rolled sleeve to protect it from the arm massage cream or oil. Then proceed as follows:

1   Cleanse both of the client's hands by wiping them over with cotton wool soaked in surgical spirit. While doing so, examine hands and nails for any contra-indications.
2   Remove existing nail enamel with varnish remover. In order to avoid damaging your own nail enamel, you should either hold the remover-soaked cotton wool between the first and second finger as low as the level of the middle phalangeal joint, well away from your own nails, or use a cotton bud soaked in remover. It many be necessary to use both. (Figure 11.) All existing enamel should be completely removed before proceeding any further. (Figure 12.)
3   Taking the client's right hand, commence shaping and reducing the length of nail using the finer side of the emery board. (Figure 13.) Always ensure that it is a new and unused board for each client. It is also a good idea that the client be made aware of this. Hygiene is like Justice – not only must it be done, but it must be seen to be done!

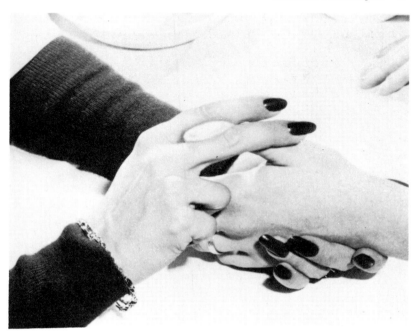

11 *Remove old varnish with cotton wool soaked in varnish remover. Hold cotton wool between fingers to avoid damage to own nail enamel*

12 *Remove enamal stubbornly clinging around edges of nail and underside using a cotton bud or cotton wool wrapped around an orange stick then soak in varnish remover*

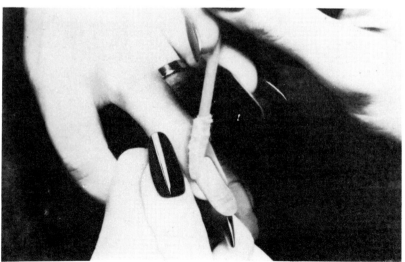

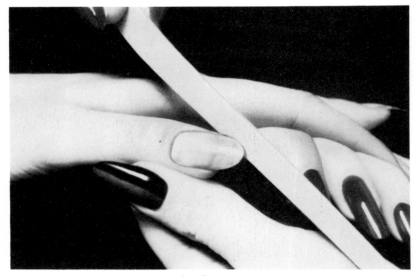

13 *File nails using finer side of emery board. Hold board under nail to bevel edge. Don't saw to and fro because this generates heat which can dry out nail and cause flaking. Just a few gentle strokes from edge to centre of nail*

14 *Apply cuticle cream around cuticle using orange stick*

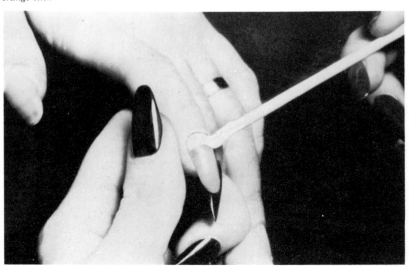

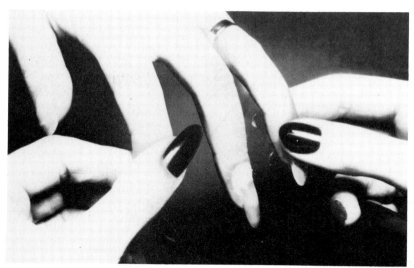

15 *Massage cuticle cream into cuticles and around the nail*

At the completion of the manicure it is advisable to break the emery board and throw it in the bin, thus preventing it from being inadvertently used on another client. This reduces the risk of any cross-infection from one client to another.

The shape of the nail should be determined by asking the client how long she wants them left and if the shape and condition of the nails is suitable (see section on nail shapes and shaping). It is pointless attempting to retain very long nails if the nail is soft and splitting or if the client does very physical work with detergents and other damaging materials or refuses to wear rubber gloves.

4 Apply cuticle softening cream or oil around the cuticles rubbing well into the cuticles with small rotary movements of the thumbs. (Figures 14 and 15.)

5 Place right hand in warm water containing either a solution of water and soft soap or water containing a special manicure 'pill' which is available. Ensure that the water container is placed safely so that the contents cannot spill on to the client's clothing. A good non-spillable shaped pot is now on the market. (Figure 16; see also section on equipment.)

6   Repeat steps 3 and 4 to client's left hand.

7   Remove right hand from water and wrap in a small, warm hand towel. Move water to client's left hand side and immerse left hand in water.

8   Unwrap right hand and apply cuticle remover to cuticles with cotton bud or orange stick wrapped with cotton wool. Gently ease back the softened cuticles with a rubber hoof stick. Great care should be taken that all treatments around the cuticle area should be as gentle as possible in order to avoid permanently damaging the very delicate matrix from which the nail is growing. If the cuticle is still adhering to the nail plate then gently scrape it away with the cuticle knife. The cuticle knife should be held so that the blade is flat against the nail surface and should be worked in small circular movements over the nail plate. At no time should it ever be used with any force to dig or poke at the cuticles. If any stubborn shreds of cuticle remain or a torn shred still hangs on, the cuticle nippers should be used. However, the practice of completely paring away the whole of the cuticle with either scissors or nippers should be avoided as this only increases the regrowth and strength of the cuticle. Remove all remnants of cuticle by wiping the area with a cotton bud soaked in cuticle remover. (Figure 17.)

9   Remove left hand from water and repeat step 8 on the left hand.

10 Commencing with the right hand, then the left, perform the massage routine which is detailed later in this chapter. As the massage routine takes about 20 minutes, ten minutes on each hand, adequate time should be allowed for this when booking the appointment. When the client is in a hurry then this step can be omitted, but the treatment is much more effective when it is left in the routine. (Figure 18.)

11 Remove massage cream or oil from the nail plates with cotton wool soaked in varnish remover and prepare hands for the application of varnish.

12 Check that no fine 'fringes' of nail have been left around the free edge after filing and then, using an orange stick wrapped with a fine pledgelet of cotton wool, clean out all massage material and other debris from under the nail. If the nails are stained then a light application of a dilute solution of hydrogen peroxide would help lift the stains.

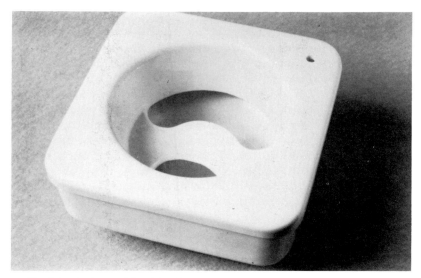

16 The Mavala 'gripper' bowl has been so designed that it can even be carried around without risk of spilling

17 Apply cuticle remover with cotton wool wrapped round orange stick. Work well in and press back cuticle

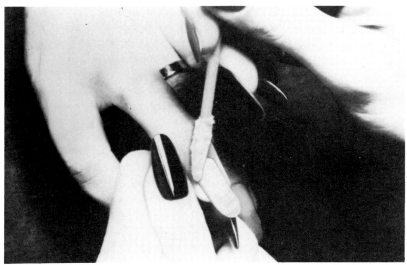

However, there is a much more effective proprietory brand of stain removing cream on the market called *Perox Chlor*. This is extremely effective and simple to use. An orange stick, wrapped in cotton wool, and then dipped in *Perox Chlor* cream should be stroked under the nails. In cases of stubborn stains, leave cream in place for a few minutes and then wash off.

This is a sensible point at which to ask the client to replace her jewellery as she may smudge the finished varnish when trying to replace rings and clip on watches, etc, at the end of the treatment. Where a client is in a hurry, it is also sensible to ask her to pay at this point as hurriedly writing a cheque or looking for her wallet can also result in a very smudged application of varnish. This, of course, should be explained to the client rather than just demand payment half way through the treatment!

13 Apply a small amount of nail buffing powder or cream to the nail surface and then buff the nails. (Figure 19.)

Buffing should be done in one direction only, never in a backwards and forwards sawing movement. This would create heat and thereby possibly damage the nail bed or matrix.

Buffing only normally takes place if the client does not intend having the nails varnished. Many clients cannot have varnish applied due to their occupations. For instance, anyone working in the food manufacturing industry, medical practitioners, nurses, dentists and many others. Also, for obvious reasons, buffing rather than nail varnish is more popular in male manicures.

14 Starting with the right hand and then the left, carefully apply a coat of clear base coat. There are many effective kinds on the market, or if the client's nails are very fragile or damaged, then apply a generous coat of a nail bonding treatment such as *Nail Magic* or Mavala nail hardener. These products, when used regularly in the manner detailed by the manufacturer, certainly strengthen and bond the type of nail which is thin and splitting in layers. (Figures 20 and 21.)

Using an orange stick with the finely pointed end dipped in nail varnish remover, lightly trace around the edge of the varnish in the cuticle area to ensure that the application of varnish has a neat edge to it. This should be done gently and

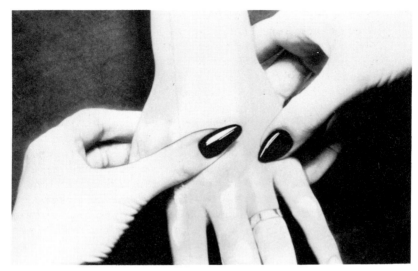

18 *Hand massage improves capillary circula-tion and generates a feeling of wellbeing*

19 *Using a buffer produces a smoother nail surface, helps to flatten unsightly ridges*

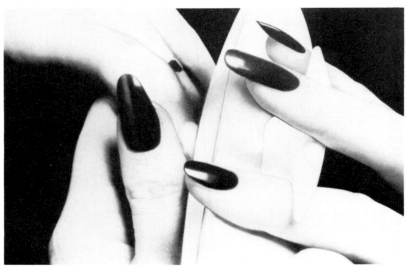

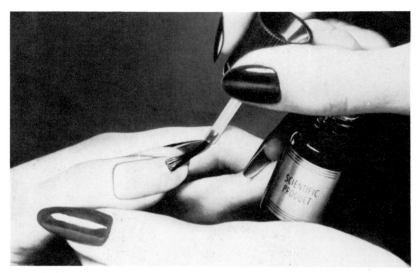

20 *Nails that crack, split or break easily benefit from an application of nail hardener – applied once a week*

21 *An application of base coat prevents colour penetrating the nail and staining the nail bed permanently*

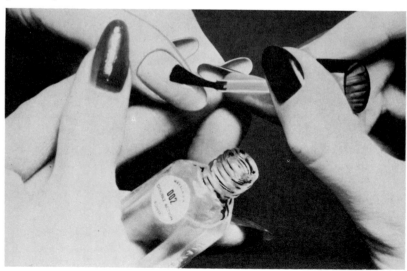

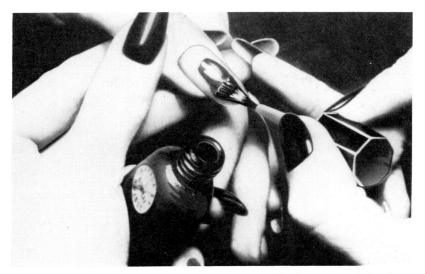

22 *Colour should be applied first with a stroke in the centre of the nail, then at the base of the nail, and finally filling in round the edges. Two coats usually suffice*

with great skill, otherwise the whole application of colour could be ruined. However, when performed correctly it gives a very neat and professional finish to the varnish.

15 Apply two thin coats of the selected nail varnish. The application should be made with as few brush strokes as possible and should easily be covered by the experienced manicurist with three strokes. (Figure 22.)

16 When dry apply a single thin coat of protective clear or top coat. If the client wishes the whole varnish can be dried by the use of a quick drying spray. Take care when using this in the confined space of a small manicure cubicle as the aerosol propellant gas can cause breathing problems with some people. If using such a spray, then be sure to ask the client to turn her head away so that she does not directly inhale the gas. Also take the same precaution yourself.

17 If time and seating space allow, ask the client to remain where she is until the varnish is completely dried. (Figure 23)

One of the most important aspects of a manicure is the correct shaping and filing of the nails. With clients who have a very short growth of nail, either from choice or because they cannot grow

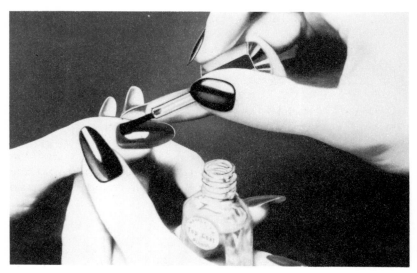

23 *An application of top coat can produce a protective finish that will survive knocks that normally chip nail enamel. With only a little care, top coat will help polish last as long as a week*

them very long, you have very little option but to file them neatly across and gently round the edges.

However, where there is a reasonable length of growth you have to decide on a length which is both acceptable to the client and realistic in relation to her lifestyle. Where you have a client who does very little with her hands all day, then provided that the nails are strong enough, the length can be quite considerable. In everyday practice however, one sees very few clients of this kind, and the majority of them are using their hands most of the day in some form of work or other.

The shape of the nails should be a pleasing almond shape, neither too pointed nor too flattened. If in doubt be guided by the shape at the cuticle end of the nail, and attempt to achieve a balanced, even look.

Using the fine side, the emery board should be held on the underside of the nail when shaping to avoid producing an irritating 'fringe' of nail tissue. The filing action should always be in strokes in one direction only. The file should never be 'sawed' backwards and forwards. The boards should always be used from sides to centre. Never file too deeply into the nail sulcus (groove) at the sides of the nail as this will produce a sharp pointed weakened nail.

Obviously you should consult the client on the length and shape she would like, but where the nails are very uneven in length it should always be suggested that they all be reduced to a uniform length. Nothing looks worse than a hand with one or two very long nails, their owner's 'pride and joy' and the rest very short as a result of breakages. You should tactfully suggest reducing them to a pleasing level. Where the nails have been subjected to very harsh conditions and they are splitting and lifting in layers, then you must firmly insist that they are worn as short as possible until the client realises that harsh chemicals and abrasives and fine nails do not go together.

Nail repairing

It is sometimes possible to repair a damaged nail if the client has only torn it partially across and if the torn piece is still present. If the nail is torn above the free edge it is better to remove the torn fragment completely and reshape the remaining nail with an emery board as breaks above the free edge are very difficult to hold in place.

However, if the tear is below the free edge, it is essential to try to refix the tear and hold it so that the very vulnerable nail bed beneath the plate does not become damaged or infected.

There are two main methods of doing this. One is to wrap the tear with tissue and special adhesive and the other is to use one of the readymade self adhesive patches sold by manicure companies.

Tissue method

Materials required
Nail adhesive glue
Absorbent tissues
Emery board
Orange stick
Nail varnish remover

Method
Remove old nail varnish and replace tear as accurately as possible. Smooth across top of tear with fine emery board if any jagged ends

are standing free. Tear a small piece of tissue slightly larger than damaged area. A torn piece blends in more easily than one with cut edges.

Paint a thin application of nail adhesive over torn area and surrounding nail plate, then quickly lay torn piece of tissue over the tear pressing into place with a soft squirrel hair painting brush. Dip the tip of your finger into nail varnish remover just to stop it sticking to the patch and mould the patch into place over the tear. When the tissue is firmly in place and completely covering the damaged area, apply another thin coat of adhesive. Smooth off any ridges or bumps with either the squirrel hair brush or your own finger moistened with varnish remover.

Allow tissue and adhesive to dry completely before applying base coat and varnish in the usual way.

This of course is only a temporary method of repair and the procedure must be repeated for every fresh application of varnish.

Self adhesive repair method
There are several self adhesive repair methods on the market, but the one described here is the *Mavala* method.

Materials required
Normal manicure equipment
Mavala nail repair kit

Method
Perform a complete manicure on both hands, but filing very gently on the finger which has the broken nail. Reduce the length of nail if possible in order to place less strain on the torn portion.

Apply base coat and two coats of colour in the normal way. When varnish is dry select nail shape from wallet as near to the size and shape of the damaged nail as possible. Lift self adhesive strip from wallet by holding it at the end with the coloured strip. Press nail repair shape firmly over damaged nail with rounded end of shape fitting firmly into cuticle area, continue to press shape on to the surface of the nail, ironing out any small air bubbles which might appear.

Trim excess adhesive shape away with a fine pair of nail scissors but leave a small margin of material around free edge of nail. Neatly tuck in this margin of adhesive around free edge of nail firmly with an orange stick. This shape will then remain in place as long as necessary but will have to be replaced if the client wishes to change her varnish colour, and also when the nail grows forward carrying the adhesive nail shape with it and thereby causing a ridge to appear. When it is necessary to replace it, the self adhesive patch lifts off quite easily.

Massage of the hand and forearm

The inclusion of a massage sequence into the manicure routine gives the whole treatment a professional touch and also relaxes the client.

The benefits of massage are:
Improves circulation
Relaxes tense muscles
Aids lymphatic drainage
Aids desquamation of top layers of dead cells
Improves absorption of creams and oils

All massage movements should be performed smoothly and rhythmically and in order to do this the hands should not stick at all. It is essential therefore that some form of medium should be used. The choice is usually between a dry substance such as talcum powder or an oil or cream.

Talc, whilst being a perfectly good medium with which to massage, does have some disadvantages. These are that it is difficult to control, the lightness of the powder makes it difficult to restrict it to the area being massaged: clients do not usually like it because of their clothes becoming soiled; it can also be very dangerous for the therapist who uses it regularly because with even the strictest of safety precautions, it is difficult not to inhale some of the powder. This would reach an unacceptable level after a very short while.

Oil is a superb medium with which to work, but like talc it is difficult to control and, without great care, it could get spilled or soil the client's clothing.

Cream as a medium therefore has to be the answer as long as it does not stick or drag on the skin, particularly on arms or legs which are hairy. The ideal formula is one in which the medium has all the characteristics of being a cream while it is in the pot and being transferred to the hands, but has such a low melting point that it takes on the consistency of oil when it comes in contact with the heat of the body. This type of cream, suitable for massage, is discussed on page 116.

Massage of the hand and arm, or indeed, any part of the human body, is best given by using the standard movements usually known as *Swedish massage*. This consists of four different types of movements, namely:

Effleurage A slow moving stroking, smoothing movement which can vary in pressure from firm and deep to a very light superficial stroking. This is the movement which is used to commence and finish a massage routine and is also used between the more vigorous movements when a calming soothing action is required.
Petrissage The compression or kneading movement. This is used to best advantage over muscles and produces a deep pumping action in the underlying tissue, thereby stimulating lymphatic drainage in the area.
Tapotement A percussion type movement which can be ·ries of brief, brisk movements given to stimulate blood lymph flow.
Frictions Usually with the ball of the thumb, these small circular pressure movements are given to loosen adhesions in underlying tissues and aid in absorption around joints.

Hand and arm massage routine

1   Holding client's left arm with your left hand just below the elbow with client's hand with the back uppermost, commence effleurage stroking from the wrist to the elbow using your right hand. Apply pressure on each stroke as the hand glides up the arm, but release pressure on the downward stroke allowing hand to simply touch the arm from elbow to wrist. Repeat this movement six times in all.
2   Slide right hand back to elbow and commence petrissage movements down outer third of lower arm. Return hand to elbow and repeat movements to central third of lower arm. Return to elbow and repeat movements to inner third of lower arm.
3   Repeat movement one, ie six effleurage from wrist to elbow.
4   Turn client's arm so that the palm is facing upwards. Change hands by supporting client's left arm with your right hand

and repeat both movements one and two giving effleurage and petrissage to the inner surface of the lower arm using your left hand.

5   Using thumbs of both hand give thumb frictions over carpal area.

6   Slide to palmar area. Using thumbs of both hands give alternate deep thumb strokes over both the thenar and the hypothenar eminences.

7   Place client's elbow on table and raise hand away from table. Link your fingers with client's whilst steadying her arm at the elbow with other hand. Gently rotate the carpal joints using the intertwined fingers. Rotate firstly clockwise, then anti-clockwise. If the client is suffering from any arthritic condition or finds this uncomfortable, this movement should be avoided.

8   Return hand to table and place palm downwards. Using the thumbs of both hands give small rotary frictions firstly all over the carpals then working down between the shafts of the metacarpals working from carpals to metacarpo-phalangeal joints with the return movement being a deep effleurage stroke.

9   Continue using a similar type of movement, but this time using the thumb and first finger, working down the length of each finger using a deep effleurage to return to joint.

10 Complete massage routine by giving six effleurage strokes over back of hand up to elbow, finishing on the last stroke at the elbow and giving a firm press before removing the hands. Remove massage cream from the arm and hand using cotton wool soaked in eau de Cologne. Surgical spirit can be used, but costing only about the same price, eau de Cologne just adds that little touch of luxury which clients appreciate so much.

Manicures for men

The ever increasing popularity of manicure treatments for men is reflected in the growth of manicure facilities being offered by very many male hairdressing establishments, health clubs, gymnasia, etc. Obviously the basic routine remains the same with just a few variations. Some men like the idea of wearing a clear gloss coat of varnish, but the majority prefer the nails to be well buffered and naturally shining rather than gloss varnished.

Nail staining and stubborn deposits under the nails of such materials as paint or car and diesel oil present more of a problem. This can be overcome by applying a stain remover such as *Perox Chlor* to a small nail brush and brushing under the nails after the initial soaking.

It is a good idea to stock a retail size of such a stain remover as most male clients are interested in maintaining the appearance of their hands and nails once they have been manicured.

Hot oil manicure

The majority of clients who attend the salon for manicure treatments are usually very conscious of the appearance of their hands and will co-operate very much with the manicurist by looking after their hands and nails while at home. Occasionally, however, one encounters badly neglected hands and nails with the skin of both the hands and the cuticle areas very dry, horny and broken. These are usually clients who work very hard manually or have spent some years doing very little other than hard housework. Usually they have not been aware of the damage this type of work can do if rubber gloves and barrier creams are not used to prevent it.

The hands would probably continue to be so abused if it were not for some special occasion, such as the wedding of a daughter, or the coming of a new grandchild to be cuddled and played with, that makes the client aware of her badly neglected hands. The manicurist is then expected to work miracles and transform the hands in one treatment!

Quite obviously this cannot be done, but a programme of intensive care can be started by the manicurist with a great emphasis being placed on home care. The client usually responds very well and becomes quite a good customer. To give the maximum amount of improvement in the initial stages one needs to commence a course of treatments using hot oils.

Materials required
All the normal manicure equipment
Electrically heated oil container
Jasmine, olive or any good plant oil

Method
File and shape the nails in the usual way.
If nails are splitting and flaking off in layers due to repeated immersion in strong detergents, file gently but advise the client that the nails are best kept as short as possible until the splits and tears are gone.
Apply cuticle oil around cuticles and massage well into skin.
The oil heater should have been set ready before the manicure commenced, with the jasmine or almond oil heating in the container. If such a heater is not available, pour some oil into an ordinary glass basin, preferably *Pyrex*, and stand this to heat up in a bowl of hot water. Never put the oil directly over the heat, always in a bath of water, otherwise a fire may occur.
Check that it is warm, but not too hot, then immerse the client's whole hand in the oil. Leave for approximately 10 to 15 minutes each hand.
After removing from the oil, dry carefully on tissues and continue with the manicure. However, the cuticle should be very gently worked on *without* the use of a cuticle remover. The chemical composition of cuticle remover is such that it has a very drying effect on the cuticles. Under normal circumstances, and used sparingly, this does not have any ill effects on the surrounding tissues, but in the case of badly dried and neglected cuticles, it should not be used.
Repeat these treatments weekly until a marked improvement is noticed, then continue with regular normal manicures.

Paraffin wax baths

Materials required
Paraffin wax heater and wax
Aluminium foil
Warm towels
This treatment can be given to hands or feet. It is most beneficial, not only to the skin, but the heat has a soothing and relaxing effect on tense or damaged muscles and ligaments as well as capsular joints and bones. It brings a relief from pain, probably only temporary, for anyone suffering from arthritic conditions of the hands or feet.

Method

Set wax heater to warm up with wax in the inner bath. With the electrical heaters the thermostat raises the wax to the correct temperature and maintains it at that level so that there is no danger of the client being burned by immersing the foot or hand in too hot a wax. However, if the treatment is being given by heating the wax independently over a water bath, great care should be taken to ensure that the wax does not become too hot.

Carry out a normal manicure or pedicure to the completion of the massage.

After checking that the wax is cool enough, submerge the hand or foot in the wax and remove, still holding it over the wax bath for any drips of molten wax to drop back into the container. The thin layer of wax that remains on the limb will be seen to be cooling slightly and hardening; when this is noticed, replace the hand or foot in the bath again and remove quickly. This action should be repeated four or five times so that the hand or foot is completely coated with four or five thin layers of wax.

Still keeping the hand or foot over the bath to catch any drips, take a piece of aluminium foil large enough to encase completely the hand or foot and wrap the limb in it. This in turn is then wrapped with pre-heated towels and set to rest for approximately 15 minutes. One limb should be done straight after the other so that the wax heater can then be moved to safety away from the working area. If there is any accidental spillage of this wax on to a carpeted area, leave it to dry. Then take a large thick pad of absorbent tissue, bed roll, or kitchen paper, place it over the wax and iron the area with a warm clothes iron. This will lift the wax and draw it into the absorbent paper. It may be necessary to repeat the process with several thick layers of paper, but if persevered with, the wax does finally lift completely from the carpet. Incidentally, this can also be done to remove spillages of all types of depilatory waxes.

After approximately 15 minutes resting time, remove towels and foil and peel off the paraffin wax. Dispose of the wax immediately. Do not be tempted to re-use it, as it will be full of perspiration and debris from the client's skin.

Wipe the skin with a soothing wipe of eau de Cologne and continue manicure or pedicure in the normal way.

Benefits
  Aids absorption of creams and oils
  Softens dried and horny skin
  Relieves aching and strained muscles
  Improves circulation and gives temporary relief from aching
  joints and arthritic conditions

Artificial nail techniques

No modern book on manicure would be complete without a
section on the special techniques of applying artificial nails.
However, it is a specialised art in itself and demands a great deal of
skill and acquired expertise if the nail is to look at all natural.

There are many different methods in use ranging from the
ready to use pre-formed stick-on nails to the build-on, sculpturing
methods of applying high strength acrylic materials. Continuing
research and development in this field results in new techniques
being evolved almost daily. This is good for the profession as it
means that if the therapist is prepared to keep up with the latest
techniques then she can offer her clients the best possible service.

To the beginner however the bewildering array of 'systems' can
be very confusing, but the best advice one can offer is to suggest
that the beginner attends one of the many excellent courses that
are arranged by either the manufacturer of the product or their
UK agents, and masters their techniques – possibly perfecting
these acquired skills with experiments and research of ones own.

Many clients are interested in this service but, unfortunately,
not all of them have nails or occupations which suit artificial nails.

The contra-indications for artificial nails are the same as for any
other manicuring techniques, but should stress the following:

1 Never on nails which are thin, delicate or unhealthy looking in
   any way.
2 They should not be applied if the cuticles or surrounding soft
   tissue is in any way infected, damaged, cut, bruised or torn
3 Artificial nails, particularly the sculptured, build-on type
   should never be applied where the client has an occupation
   which may result in the artificial nail being subjected to strong
   chemicals which could penetrate around the edges of the nails
   and cause deterioration of the natural tissues.
4 They should not be applied if the client intends subjecting

them to strong work which may result in them being caught and torn. Invariably the high strength artificial nail holds firm under such stress, but the natural nail beneath gets torn instead.

Artificial nails can be used for:
1   Improving the appearance of the hands where the client finds it very difficult to grow her own nails to any length because they break or tear.
2   Curing the client of nail-biting. This is providing that the nail-biting has not resulted in permanent damage to the natural nail or the nail-bed or cuticles.
3   Matching up one or two broken nails to the length and shape of the client's natural nails.
4   For a special occasion such as a wedding or similar event where the client wishes to appear well-groomed particularly in photographs.

When the nails are intended to be worn for any length of time and on a regular basis, the manicurist should be realistic about the length of the nail that she designs. Many sets of artificial nails come to grief unnecessarily because they have been designed purely for appearance sake without taking into account the client's habits and occupation. Very few women today do nothing at all, so a quick discussion on the client's working day will dictate the style and length of nail. Anyone who uses a keyboard such as a typist, VDU operator or a supermarket till will not be able to work with some of the longer style nails. A young mum with children would find them decidedly dangerous and even the most glamorous of models may find the very long nails a positive hazard when trying to fasten and unfasten buttons and zips during a fast moving, quick change fashion show! The moral being – if you want the nails to last and your reputation to stay intact – be realistic!

Nail sculpturing

By far the most popular method of applying artificial nails is the technique of building and sculpting artificial nails using high tensile acrylic materials or organic polymer resins. The materials usually consist of a powder and liquid which are freshly mixed for each set of nails and applied immediately.

As stated before, there are many systems and methods of application so the following instructions are a general guide and an amalgam of the more popular techniques.

Preparation of nails
The nails are manicured in the usual way until the stage is reached at which the base coat would normally be applied. Special attention should be given to ensure that the cuticles have been softened and eased back neatly without any traces adhering to the nail plate as this would spoil the appearance of the finished nails. The nails should then be washed and brushed with a nail brush to remove all traces of cuticle remover or massage cream. The nail is then finally wiped over with a trace of varnish remover to ensure that no oil or grease is present. (Figures 24, 25 and 26.)

Material needed
Pure squirrel or sable brushes
Organic polymer powder
Organic polymer resin liquid
Two small plastic containers for holding ingredients
Foil nail formers in varying shapes and sizes (some systems use
    disposable formers, others re-usable ones)

24 *Push up cuticle to remove cuticle membrane*

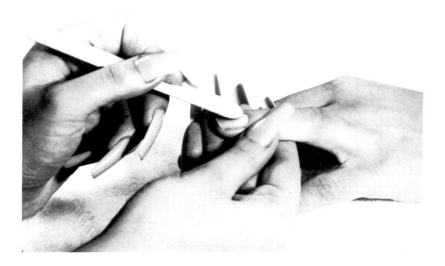

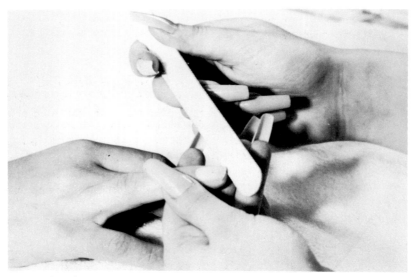

25 *Even free edge*

26 *Roughen surface of nail gently to remove shine and bacteria, and also sterilize nail with fresh nail*

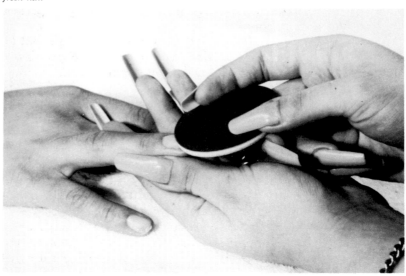

Liquid brush cleanser
Liquid anti-bacterial primer

Routine
1   Prepare nail plate surface by roughening the surface all over
    with a fine emery board to remove the natural oil and prepare
    the surface for a better bonding between the artificial and
    natural nail. Early systems roughened the nail with a drill or
    rough emery to a very great depth which not only caused
    discomfort, but often damaged the nail plate permanently.
    This ideas has been superceded by the development of the
    organic polymer resins which do not need such a rough
    surface to form a retention bond. With the present methods
    it is sufficient only to remove the natural oil and natural
    shine.
2   Remove all traces of dust from the nail and apply a coat of
    quick drying anti-bacterial primer. (Figure 27.) Allow to dry.
    This is essential to clear the nail of any bacteria which might
    be present.
3   Select a foil nail shape or former which corresponds with the
    shape and size of the free edge of the natural nail. Place the
    foil former on the finger, under the free edge of the natural
    nail, wrapping and moulding the foil shape around the tip of
    the finger so that it remains firmly in place whilst building is
    taking place. (figure 28.)
       Small amounts of the powder and the liquid should be
    already prepared in the small containers. The powder is
    normally a slightly tinted shade, but a more recent develop-
    ment of using two shade powders, a tinted one for the body
    of the nail and a whiter one for the tip is very popular. Using
    this system it will be necessary to prepare the two coloured
    powders in the same way.
4   Apply one coat of base primer, allow to dry completely
    before applying second coat. Allow to dry.
5   Using a very clean sable brush, dip it into the liquid and
    withdraw, drawing brush against side of container to remove
    excess liquid. (Figure 29.)
6   Dip the tip of the brush containing the small amount of
    liquid into the powder and roll the tip of the brush in the
    powder to trace the letter 'O'. This action results in the tip of
    the brush picking up a small ball of the material. (Where a

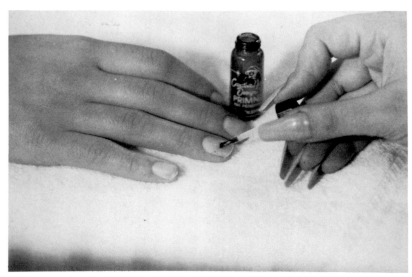

27 *Apply primer to nail to ensure chemical bonding of nail product*

28 *Fit aluminium form*

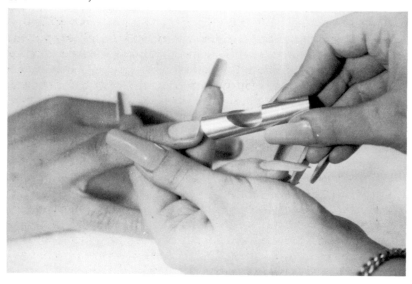

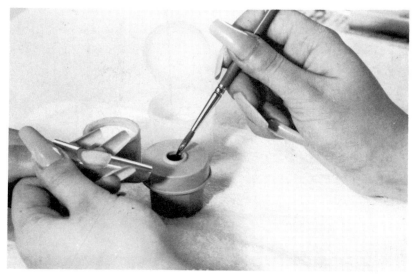

29 *Moisten brush with nail liquid*

different colour tip powder is being used, this first application should be of the lighter, tip powder.)

7   Quickly place the ball of material which has formed on the brush in the centre of the seam where the free edge of the nail meets the foil nail former. Rotate the brush so that the ball of material rolls off the brush and then working quickly with as few movements as possible press the ball into the desired shape using the base rather than the tip of the hair of the brush. (Figure 30.) Spread the material out to the desired length of nail tip, brushing and moulding with the brush.

8   Dip brush into brush cleaning liquid to remove any traces of material. Dry on a tissue.

9   Dip brush into active liquid and this time pick a small ball of the shaded nail body powder. Place ball of material approximately one third of the way down the nail between the free edge and the lunula. Spread and mould this ball of material as before, working back upwards towards the free edge. As the material is being formed and spread evenly all over the surface of the nail, great care should be taken that the material covers all of the nail yet does not come into contact with the soft tissue of the cuticle or nail sulcus.

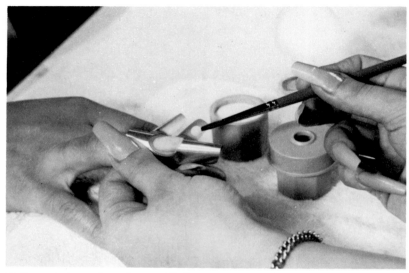

30 *Rotate in tip powder to form small ball*

31 *Pat and press to shape using body of brush.*
To form a perfect looking nail tip, continue with
clear powder and liquid to cover and blend with
natural nail

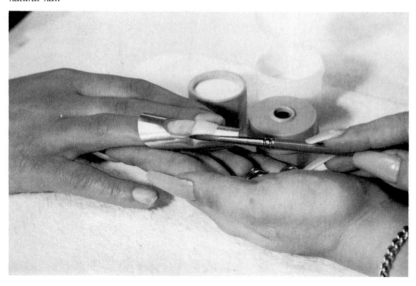

10 The third application of the material should be prepared in the same manner as the two former, except in this application the mix is much wetter. This means that more fluid and less powder should be taken up and mixed together. The resulting much softer, moister ball of material should be placed a small distance from the lunula and quickly worked backwards and outwards using the body of the brush. Using the brush in this very wet manner means that any bumps or ridges in the material can be softened and smoothed out, thus leaving the nail with little or no finishing filing to be done. (Figure 31.)
11 This nail should be left to dry completely and work can begin on another nail while this is drying. The nails are fully hardened when you can hear a dry crisp clicking sound on tapping the artificial nail.
12 On ensuring that the nail is emitting the correct sound when tapped, gently remove foil former taking care not to bend the new nail in any way. The nail is then ready for filing and shaping to the desired length and shape, firstly with a rough emery and then with varying grades of finer emery boards. (Figure 32.) Finally buff the nails with the special buffing tool until the entire surface is smooth and a shine starts to form. (Figure 33 and 34.)
13 Apply a good cuticle oil not only to the surface of the artificial nail, but also to the cuticle and surrounding soft tissue. (Figure 35.)
14 Wash and dry nail thoroughly and repeat procedures on all other nails.
15 When all nails are complete apply base coat, varnish coat and top coat exactly as one would in the normal manicure. (Figure 36.)

With this new type polymer resin, the nail can be built up to whatever thickness desired, and quite obviously the thinner the better for appearance sake, but one requires a certain amount of depth for strength.

If the finished nail is too thick it may be necessary to reduce the thickness with an electric nail drill.

For safety reasons, anyone using such a drill should always wear a face mask to limit the amount of dust inhaled.

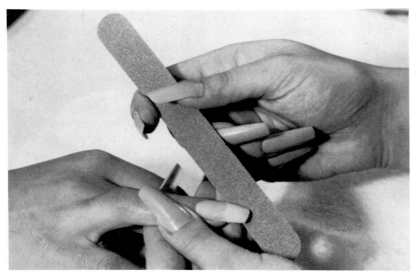

32 *The nail is now set after 3–5 minutes – shape free edge*

33 *Buff entire nail to smooth*

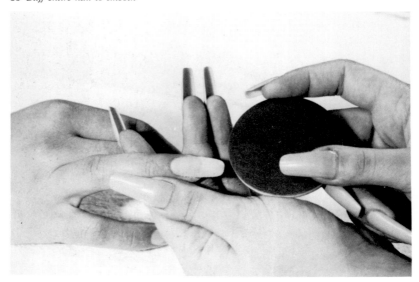

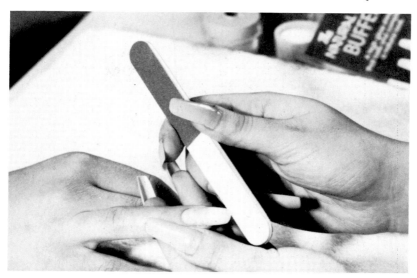

34 *Buff to a high gloss with natural nail buffer*

35 *Condition with rich cuticle oil*

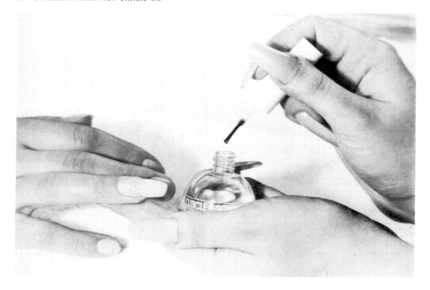

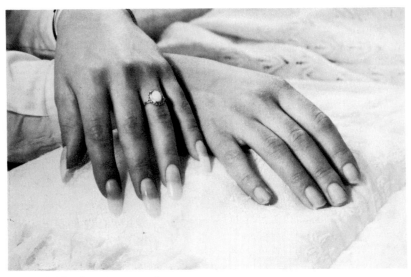

36 *Finished hand can be compared to previous
short, bitten, or broken nails!*

Nail covering
This method of nail sculpturing can be used simply to reinforce or repair one or two nails which have become torn, usually below the free edge. In this instance the procedure is the same except that you would not require the foil former and the nail would not be extended in length.

Fill-ins
As the natural nail grows so the artificial nail appears to grow away from the lower edge around the cuticle, leaving an unsightly gap. This must be attended to on a regular basis, so the client is instructed to return in approximately two to three weeks for a check-up. The procedure on a 'fill-in' session is as follows:

1   Prepare nails by removing all polish and cleanse nail by brushing with soapy water and nail brush.
2   Apply cuticle remover to cuticle and treat in the normal manner, easing them back gently. Clip away any thin or crumbling and loose particles of the artificial nail material. Take care not to damage the natural nail or the cuticles during this operation.

3   Gently roughen the new area of natural nail with an emery board.

4   Repeat the same procedure as for the original nail build, ensuring that first the anti-bacterial primer is used, then the ordinary primer, then the polymer resin itself.

5   When dry shape and file in the former manner, finishing with buffing and re-lacquering with coloured varnish.

As with all skills which require deftness and precision combined with speed, the art of nail sculpting needs careful practice before one can build these nails with the degree of professional competency needed. However, it is surprising how quickly one acquires the deftness if confident to try.

The main criticism of nail sculpting seems to be that the early methods nearly all employed the use of pre-formed moulds which made the nails look very thick and chunky. Another valid criticism is that many nail sculpting artists make them too long, once again making them vulnerable to wear and tear. This in turn makes them unpopular with the clients.

Those who make them a realistic length and have perfected the technique of making them as thin as a normal nail certainly gain a wonderful reputation and are never short of willing clients.

Detachable artificial nails

Sets of detachable artificial nails are available, made either of plastic or nylon, which can look quite realistic if the client wishes to wear them for only one special occasion and cannot wear the sculpted nail. This type of artificial nail which is held in place by a special adhesive can only be worn for short durations and should never be worn for longer than 48 hours at a time.

Method of Application

1   Manicure client's hands up to the point at which one would normally apply base coat.

2   Roughen the client's nails slightly with a fine emery. As with the nail sculpting, the up-to-date material used as a fixative does not require the natural nail to be too deeply roughened.

3   These attractive sets of nails come in a variety of shapes and sizes and will obviously look more natural if the size and shape selected follow the natural shape of the client's own nails,

although longer. If all the sets appear to be too long, they can be reduced in length by trimming them with ordinary nail clippers or scissors and then filing them smooth. If the shape and convexity of the nail is not quite right, thereby causing the shape not to fit the natural nail, this can be altered by immersing the shape in warm water for a few minutes and then gently bending to the required shape. To restore its original firmness, drop the reshaped nail into cold water for a few minutes before using.

4   Apply small amounts of adhesive around the edges of the natural nail, taking care not to let the adhesive flood the cuticle area or cover the centre of the nail plate.

5   Apply a few drops of the adhesive on the inside of the nail form avoiding the area which will be the free edge tip.

6   Gently slide the bottom edge of the shape slightly under the softened cuticle, or if not possible, up as near to the cuticle as possible. Allow the nail shape to flatten gently against the natural nail. Hold firmly in place for a few minutes for the adhesive to form a bond.

7   Carefully clean away any adhesive that has oozed out around the edge or under the tip.

8   Allow the artificial nails to dry completely before completing the treatment by applying the normal coats of varnish.

The client should be warned to treat the nails very gently until they are completely set. She should also be advised that they are not suitable for wearing and doing manual work. Repeatedly immersing them in very hot water may loosen the adhesive. Most manufacturers insist that they should only be worn for a maximum length of 48 hours and of course the normal contra-indications to manicure apply to the application of this style of artificial nail. Most of the adhesives are inflammable so great care should be taken in the cubicle when using them. Care should be taken that only acetone-free varnish removers are used on plastic nails.

Nail tips

Yet another method of artificially giving a client the appearance of having long, well-manicured nails is the rather more difficult method of applying nail tips. These artificial nail tips also come in

a variety of shapes and sizes and include comprehensive instructions from the manufacturers.

Method of use

1 Manicure the hands in the normal manner up to but not
   including the application of base coat.
2 File free edge of client's natural nail in a shape to correspond
   with the lower edge of the nail tips selected. As with the nail
   sculpting, the sensible choice of a realistic length nail tip will
   certainly ensure that the tip remains firmer and in place a lot
   longer than a grossly elongated obviously false nail.
3 Using a fine emery board, roughen slightly the last 5mm of
   the natural nail.
4 Apply a tiny drop of adhesive along the groove on the convex
   edge of the nail tip.
5 Fix nail tip in place by overlapping on the free edge of the
   natural nail. Ensuring that the tip is in the correct place, hold
   firmly for a few minutes to allow adhesive to set.
6 Apply another small amount of adhesive over join, both on
   top and under nail.
7 When dry, take a fine emery board and file the seam gently so
   that a small amount of white powder appears. Apply another
   few drops of the adhesive over the white powder to form a
   bond and filler across the seam. Allow to dry and repeat
   several times.
8 File the edges of nail tip to correspond with client's natural
   nails.
9 Apply several coats of adhesive thinly over tip from seam to
   tip of extension. Allow to harden thoroughly before
   proceeding.
10 When completely dry and hard, file gently with fine emery to
   smooth out any bumps or unevenness.
11 Apply varnish in the normal way.

Tips and sculpting

A new idea to emerge from experiments carried out by a beauty
therapist is to combine the use of tips, but instead of just the
adhesive, the new technique floats over the top of the completed
tip a couple of thin applications of the organic polymer resin one
usually sculpts with. This reinforces the tips and cuts down a lot
on the time taken to build the tip using the sculpting method.

Silk wrapping

Another new innovation designed specifically to help the client whose natural nails are weak and have a tendency to splitting and layering is the use of fine silk to wrap the nail.

The technique is exactly the same as the tissue method of nail repair described in chapter 3, but instead of tissue the nails are bonded with fine layers of natural silk and a special adhesive. This gives a reinforced bonding to the natural nail surface, thereby strengthening them and protecting them.

This type of bonding however grows with the nail and needs to be replaced at frequent intervals.

Fantasy nails

Often the manicurist is called on to produce something a little different from the normal manicure, especially for parties and other festive occasions.

With a little practice it is quite easy to produce very attractive and complicated versions of nail varnish by cutting out shapes, ie stars, stripes, zigzags, etc, from adhesive tape. Lay these to one side whilst a normal manicure is performed and the nails lacquered in a light shade or even white. Allow this application of varnish to dry completely before gently placing on the adhesive forms. Then apply one or two coats of a darker, contrasting shade of varnish. Allow to dry, then remove shapes. This leaves the contrasting lighter shade showing through the patterned shape where the adhesive patch has been.

Many manufacturers are now producing fancy nail patches for wearing on the nails as well as glitters and sequins, etc, for decorating the nail after the last application of varnish.

The ultimate of chic and elegance in fantasy nail wear must surely go to the very well known beauty therapy lecturer who is never seen without her solid nine carat gold artificial finger nail always on the fourth finger of her left hand. On the instructions of her insurance company, a special adhesive must be used to keep it in place.

4 Pedicure treatment

Preparation of pedicure trolley for use; Pedicure techniques: nail clipping, filing, cuticle care, treatment of hard skin, enamelling nails; Massage of the lower leg and foot

Materials needed

Towels and disposable towels
Bowl, preferably square, large enough to hold solution of antiseptic in which to soak feet. Or if available, specially designed plastic foot tray (see under list of suppliers for details)
Bowl of antiseptic solution to hold instruments
Cuticle knife
Rubber hoof stick
Orange stick
Heavy duty nail clippers
Cuticle clippers
Cotton wool
Tissues

Nail files and/or emery boards
Electric emery drill (if available)
Cuticle softening oil
Cuticle remover cream or lotion
Hard skin remover cream
Massage oil or cream
Surgical spirit
Eau de Cologne
Nail varnishes, coloured and clear
Instant drying spray
Nail buffer pad
Buffing powder
Toe separators

Contra-indications to pedicure
Any infectious nail or skin condition
Black or blue nails or badly damaged nails of recent origin
An obviously shedding nail
Cuts, bruises or abrasions
Broken bones, sprains or any serious swelling of the foot, ankle or leg
Skin infections
Athletes foot, or any fungal foot infections
Ingrowing toenails (rest of foot may be treated but avoid touching nail of affected toe)
See also chapter 5

Preparation for pedicure

A pedicure should not be thought of as being simply a manicure of the feet. A good pedicure can not only please the client by the improved appearance of the feet, but can bring untold relief, comfort-wise. This in turn makes the client feel less stressed and her whole body, posture and even facial appearance can be improved

As the hands and feet perform entirely different functions, one must study the foot and the role it plays in supporting the body, and treat it accordingly.

The various studies of the theory of evolution of man have put forward the idea that the hands and feet were originally designed for the same purpose and a comparative study of the skeleton of the hand and foot will certainly support this theory. It will also be apparent however that the foot has changed and adapted in order to carry out the function it now has, that of supporting the whole body weight.

When man walked as an animal, it was on all fours and the weight distribution of the body was totally different by being shared equally between the hands and the feet. Now after millions of years, the legs and feet have developed a more specialised role and format. The bones of the leg and foot have thickened to provide a much heavier, more stable framework of support, while the bones of the forearm and hand are much lighter and more effectively weighted to provide the function that they now have, that of movement and speed.

The structure and position of the bones of the feet form a very complex subject to study, so for the purposes of the pedicurist it can be simplified by saying that the weight of the body is supported on a bone structure in the form of a tripod. The weight of the body is taken from the tibia by the talus, then is spread out evenly between the calcaneum at one point of the tripod and the metatarsal heads at the other two points of balance.

The whole structure is evenly controlled and balanced by the interaction of the longitudinal and transverse arches and a series of interwoven ligaments, tendons and muscles.

This works effectively and efficiently if the foot is used in a free-moving and unfettered manner. Visualise the bare foot of a young child as it learns to walk, and it can be seen that the whole structure of the foot is used to support the body as well as allow ease of movement. However, problems arise as one gets older and begins to encase the foot in shoes.

Research and development in the shoe industry have done a great deal towards eradicating many of the problems, but fashions still dictate, so that both male and female often abuse their feet by attempting to walk in shoes that do not give complete freedom of movement and are restrictive in one way or another.

It is this constant abuse of the feet which lead to many foot problems such as corns and callouses caused by pressure, ingrowing toenails and many others. These disorders are of course the work of the chiropodist and not the pedicurist who is mainly concerned with the appearance rather than the function of the foot. However, it is necessary for the pedicurist to recognise these problems in order to be able to advise clients to seek treatment from the chiropodist.

The tripod weight-bearing theory is often apparent by the very hard thickening of the skin on the plantar surface of the feet, both at the heel end of the foot and more frequently around the area of the metatarsal heads. These thickenings called *callouses* can often seriously impair the correct functioning of the foot, causing the person to walk awkwardly and thereby upsetting the correct balance not only of the foot but also of the whole body. This in turn can lead to aches and pains in other areas totally unrelated to the feet.

Corns are caused by the pressure of the footwear on specific parts of the foot, and can appear on the dorsal or upper surfaces of the toes as well as the plantar surfaces of both foot and toes. Occasionally soft corns appear between the toes.

A very uncomfortable and unsightly build-up of hard skin is often seen by the pedicurist. It is usually the result of certain types of footwear, mostly from the 'mule' type shoe and often from the exercise sandal. The repeated slapping of the heel cup of the shoe against the foot can cause large very thickened ridges of hard dry skin around the heels and on the sides of the feet, particularly in some specific occupations which involve repeated standing, such as hairdressing.

As with many things, prevention is better than cure, and clients should be advised to avoid wearing this type of footwear. In extreme cases where the area has become very cracked and sore, it should be suggested that the client covers the area with a very thick emollient cream, such as simple zinc and castor oil cream, and leaves it in place for some time, especially at a time when the feet could be warm and aid absorption of the emollient cream.

As the cream is rather messy it should be suggested that the client wears a pair of white tennis socks over it, possibly when going to bed. There are also many proprietory brands of cream on the market specifically designed for this purpose.

The chair
The ideal chair for giving a pedicure is obviously one designed specifically for that purpose, but in many salons one has to use or adapt whatever is available. However, it is important that the client sits in a chair which gives full support to the back and is the correct height so that the pedicurist herself is not under any strain. Therefore a chair which is slightly higher than the average is useful. If the salon has a hydraulic beauty chair, then this should be used, with either a foot rest attached to the chair or some other improvisation with the leg being supported by a stool or similar.

The client is asked to remove her footwear and stockings or tights and both bare feet are immersed in the footbath containing an antiseptic solution and soft soap. (Figure 37.)

Allow the feet to remain soaking for five minutes (this gives the pedicurist time to check her trolley and make sure that she has all she needs in the way of equipment and clean towels, etc).

A trolley for pedicures can be left made up and ready for use as long as the small instruments are kept in a steriliser until required.

Pedicure routine
Remove feet from footbath and dry on a disposable towel. (Figure 38.) Examine both feet closely for any signs of contra-indications. If none exist proceed as follows: Wrap right foot in a warm towel and set to one side (the uncovered foot gets cold very quickly). Take the left foot and place on prepared surface, either a stool covered in towels and then a disposable cover over the top or on your lap similarly covered.

1   Using heavy nail clippers, cut toe nails straight across. If not long enough to cut, simply reduce length by filing. Where sulcus (nail fold) obscures corner of nail, ease back gently with orange stick and ensure that there is no fine shard of nail remaining. This, if left, will grow forward and dig into the nail sulcus causing an 'ingrowing toenail'. Many theories have been put forward as a prevention and sometimes cure for ingrowing toenails. The most persistent of these 'cures' is that of cutting a V in the centre of the nail in order to reduce pressure and prevent the nail ingrowing. Research by eminent chiropodists has proved that this has no effect whatsoever, and only manages to cause the client a great deal of discomfort and distress due to hosiery continuously getting caught and scagged on these Vs.

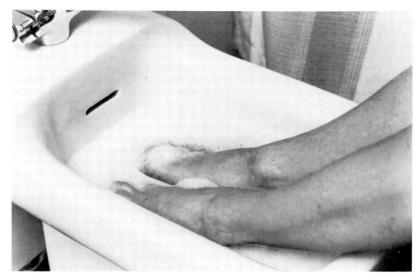

37 *A luxurious foot soak prior to Pedicure in a foot bath specially designed for the purpose*

38 *Dry feet after initial soaking with a disposable tissue and examine closely for any contraindications*

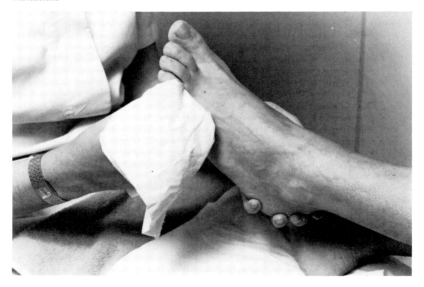

When using the nail clippers to reduce the length of the nails, avoid particles of cut nail flying into your eyes by placing the thumb of the hand which is supporting the foot over the nail being cut. (Figure 39.)

2 Finish off nails by filing first with rough emery and then finally with the smooth. (Figure 40.)

3 Apply cuticle softening oil or cream to the cuticles with an orange stick wrapped in cotton wool and return left foot to water.

Take right foot and repeat steps 1–3.

Return right foot to water.

Remove left foot from water and dry well on disposable towel.

4 Using an orange stick wrapped in cotton wool, apply a small amount of cuticle removing cream or lotion to each softened cuticle.

Using the rubber hoof stick, gently ease away any cuticle which is clinging to the nail surface. If very stubborn, use the cuticle knife with the blade held flat against the nail plate to free the cuticle and ease it back. Cuticle nippers should be used very gently at this point if any of the cuticle is torn or hanging. Carefully clear away dead skin and cuticle debris. (Figures 41 and 42.)

It is not good practice to cut away extensively the cuticle with the nippers or scissors as this tends to make the cuticle grown more profusely and both thicker and harder.

When all nails have been treated remove all traces of cuticle and cuticle removing solution by wiping the nail plates with cotton wool soaked in an antiseptic solution or surgical spirit.

5 Apply a rough skin remover cream and remove any superficial layers of dead skin by rubbing the feet with the cream. (Figures 43 and 44.)

If an electrically operated emery disc is available use this instead of the cream to gently remove any dry or hard skin from the feet. (Figure 45.) Care should be taken not to keep the disc in one area too long as this might cause discomfort.

An open blade or scalpel should not be used by the pedicurist to remove hard skin or corns.

6 Wrap left foot again in warm towel and remove right foot from water. Dry well and repeat stages 4 and 5.

The water can then be removed from the area at this time and the pedicure continues as follows.

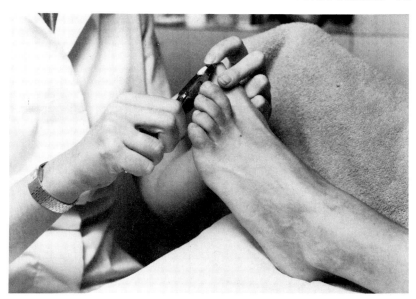

39 *Cutting toe nails with the heavy duty nail clippers. Note the index finger held lightly over* the clipping action to prevent the nail clippings from flying into the eyes

40 *Neaten the clipped nails by filing with first the rough, then the smooth emery board*

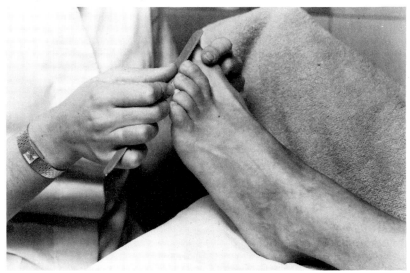

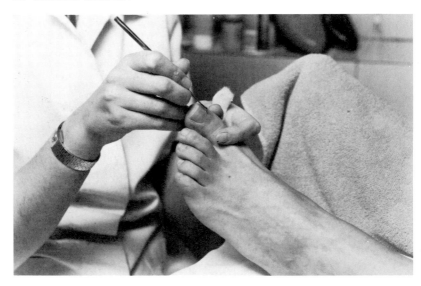

41 Carefully clear away lifted cuticle and dead skin debris from the nail plate and sulcus

42 Loosen clinging cuticles with the cuticle knife by using it with the blade held flat against the nail plate

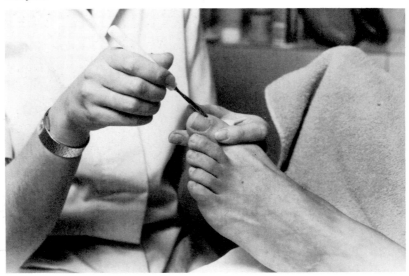

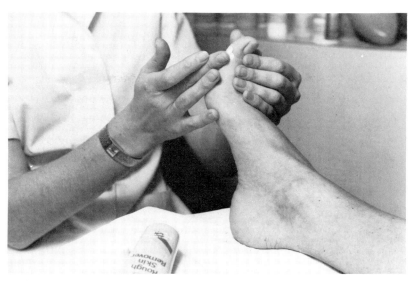

43 *Removing hard skin with a hard skin removing cream*

44 *Removing hard skin with an electrically powered emery disc. This should be kept moving to avoid trimming too deeply in one area*

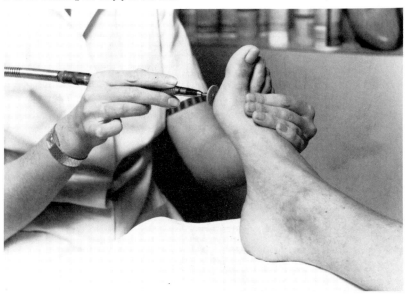

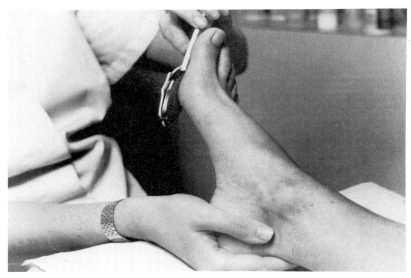

45 *Remove hard skin on plantar surface of foot with a hard skin removing implement, never with a scalpel or knife*

46 *Dust the feet lightly with a deoderising talcum or foot powder*

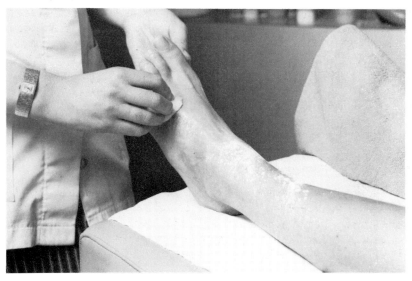

7 Apply massage medium and perform massage of foot and lower leg. A massage routine suitable for this purpose is detailed on page 98.

Remove any remaining massage cream or oil from the leg and foot by wiping with a pad of cotton wool soaked in eau de Colongne. This gives a more luxurious touch to the treatment and is equally as effective as surgical spirit.

8 Gently dust between the toes with talcum powder. (Figure 46.) Repeat steps 7 and 8 to other foot and then continue.

9 As toes sometimes touch or overlap, it is necessary to separate them in some way before varnish can be applied to the nails.

There are foam rubber moulds available for this purpose but the question of hygiene arises if this type of appliance is used for successive clients. The toe moulds should be scrubbed with a nail brush in running water and then placed in the steriliser for at least one hour.

Many therapists find it easier and safer to use a disposable method of separating the toes. This can be done by rolling up little 'sausages' of cotton wool and placing between the toes. Alternatively, as cotton wool is becoming quite expensive, ordinary tissues can be folded and interwoven between the toes (see figure 47.). This can then be disposed of in the normal way at the end of the treatment.

Before varnishing, a refreshing spray can be used on legs and feet. (Figure 48.) Apply one base coat. Follow by two coats of coloured varnish as with manicure. (Figure 49.) If the client does not wish to wear nail varnish on the toes, finish off the pedicure by applying a small amount of buffing powder to each nail and buffing gently with the nail buffer. This should be used in one direction only, never in a backwards and forwards movement as this creates heat in the nail plate.

Massage of the lower leg and foot

The pedicurist does not usually have time to perform a detailed massage of the lower leg and foot as would be the case if the client were having a full body massage. However, certain essential movements have been taken from the main routine and others added to give the pedicurist a massage routine which will be equally effective and beneficial.

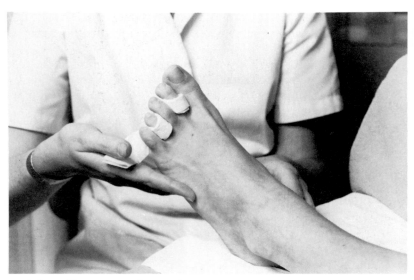

47 *A disposable tissue woven between the toes keeps them apart so that they do not touch or overlap when applying varnish. More hygenic than rubber toe separators*

48 *A refreshing spray used on both feet and legs adds a touch of luxury to a pedicure*

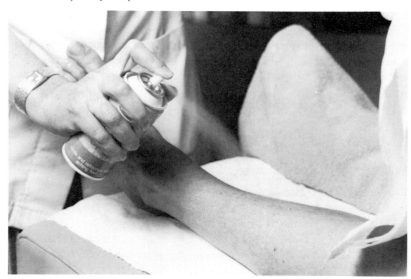

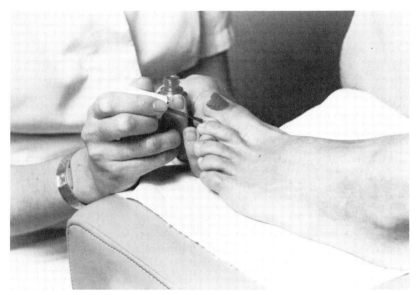

49 *Carefully apply a coat of nail varnish to
match the finger nails*

The principal benefits of massage are:
Relaxes the client
Aids desquamation of superfluous dead cells from the skin's
    surface
Relaxes and tones muscles, thereby aiding blood and lymph flow
Aids the absorption of creams or oils by the creation of heat in the
    tissues

The choice of massage material, ie whether to use powder,
cream or oil, depends largely on the personal preference of both
the pedicurist and the client. All three mediums are equally
suitable, but do have some disadvantages.

Powder is often rejected as it can make a mess of client's
clothing and carpeted working areas. It is also not so good for a
pedicurist who spends all day working on the feet as she would
obviously inhale large quantities of powder which might cause
upper respiratory infections.

Oil as a medium is very effective but can sometimes soil
clothing and carpets because of its runny consistency.

Creams can sometimes cause a 'drag' on the skin, particularly if the client is hairy. This problem can be overcome by using a massage cream which has all the consistencies and properties of a cream while in the jar and on the spatula, but which melts to an oil on contact with the skin's surface. Details of such a cream are given at the end of the book under the list of suppliers.

Massage routine

1   Six deep effleurage movements from base of toes on dorsal surface of foot, up over ankle area to patella, slide around into popliteal space and then slide lightly down back of leg, around malleolus and around to dorsal surface of foot again. On final movement stay in popliteal space. (Figure 50.)
2   Six digital stroking to popliteal space.
3   Slide hands to base of gastrocnemius muscle and commence double handed wringing movement from insertion to origin. Repeat three times. (Figure 51.)
4   Apply petrissage to belly of gastrocnemius by gently squeezing muscle with one hand and dropping it into the other. Repeat three times.
5   Six deep effleurage to back of lower leg from Achilles tendon to popliteal space.
6   Return hands to front of leg and slide to patella. Using the thenar eminence at the base of the thumb, give pressure movements down the length of the tibialis anterior and the underlying muscles.
7   Deep effleurage up shin to patella and repeat last movement six times.
8   Slide hands down to tarsal region. Using the thumbs of each hand make a series of kneading movements along the path of the metatarsals from the tarsals to the metatarso-phalangeal joints returning to the starting point by a deep sliding, stroking movement and then continuing until the whole of the dorsal surface has been covered. (Figure 52.)
9   Thumb stroke the plantar surface of the foot commencing at the base of the toes and continuing in a 'sawing' movement until the ball of the heel is reached. This movement sounds as though it would cause great discomfort to the client by 'tickling' but if the foot is held firmly by the fingers on the dorsal surface and the thumbs are used very firmly on the

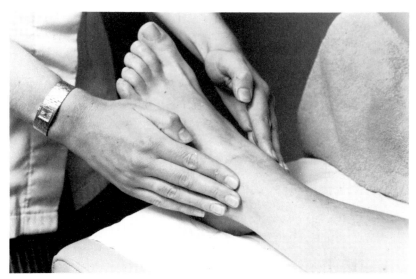

50 *Commence massage with a soothing effleurage movement*

51 *The return stroke back down the leg in effleurage is always with very light pressure*

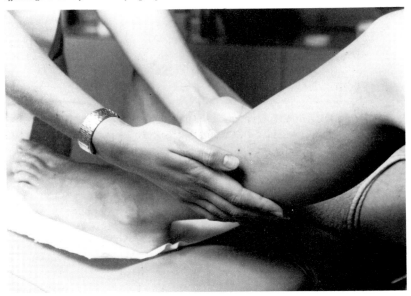

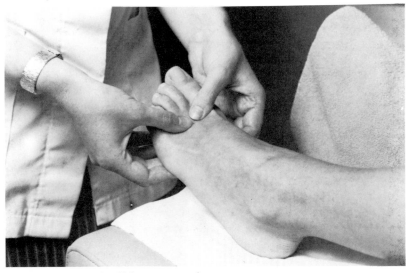

52 *Thumb frictions should be given over the metatarsal-phalangeal joints*

    plantar surface, it creates a soothing movement rather than tickling.

10   Return to dorsal surface and give slow smooth effleurage movements from base of toes to ankles.

11   Separate the hands and do digital stroking around the malleolei.

12   Finish massage by six effleurage strokes from base of toes as in movement no 1.

    Remove massage medium with a pad of cotton wool soaked in eau de Cologne or surgical spirit.

    Repeat whole of massage routine to other leg.

    Continue with pedicure routine.

5 Skin and nail disorders

Recognition of skin and nail disorders that contra-indicate manicure and pedicure; Recognition of infectious conditions which should be referred to a GP or State Registered Chiropodist; Hygiene in treatments, treatment areas and sterilisation of equipment; Dangers of cross-infections

There are many disorders and irregularities of both skin and nail which are encountered by the manicurist/pedicurist. Some contra-indicate treatment, but there are also those which do not present any problems if treated with care.

It is essential to learn how to distinguish between the safe and the contra-indicated problems, and also how to decline, politely but firmly, from working on hands or feet which have contra-indications. Where one exists which needs medical treatment the therapist should tactfully advise the client to seek help without alarming or appearing to be 'bullying' her. However, one should insist that the client should consult either her own GP or a State Registered Chiropodist.

Nail disorders

Furrows

These are either transverse or longitudinal and may develop in the nail for a variety of reasons. They can be the result of a systemic illness, but can also be cause by damage to the cells of the matrix from which the nail plate grows. Often a too-vigorous manicure either by the client or manicurist can result in this type of irregularity. Often they are the result of a childhood injury.

Beau's lines

These are deep transverse depressions in the nail plate associated with a serious illness. They are often seen following such childhood ailments as mumps and measles, but in mature adults as a result of coronary thrombosis or pneumonia. They will usually grow out unless the illness caused a permanent damage to the cellular structure of the matrix, in which case they will always be present. In really severe cases the nail sheds and continues to shed due to the damaged matrix.

Leukonychia

White patches or sometimes stripes in the nail. A common explanation often quoted is that the person is lacking in calcium in the body. There does not appear to be any evidence to support this theory whatsoever. The main reason appears to be incomplete keratinisation of some of the cells in the formation of the nail plate. These usually get smaller as the patch moves its way up the nail. Also this can, once again, be the result of a rough manicuring technique.

Pterygium

An abnormally thick and persistent growth of the cuticle which appears to grow up the nail with the nail plate. Sometimes this is the result of very poor peripheral circulation, but in many cases there does not appear to be any obvious reason for this sudden growth. It must be treated with great care and the client must be instructed on how to keep the nail plate free from the pterygium between visits. Pterygium will sometimes also affect the area under the free edge of the nail with a seemingly thick outgrowth of the hyponychium. This is extremely uncomfortable and should be gently eased back with a rubber hoof stick.

Onychosis

This is a general term given to any disease of the nail.

Onycholysis

One of the most frequently seen disorders of the nail is a shedding nail. This can occur due to a knock or a blow of some description. A common one is shutting the hand in the car door, which usually results in the middle finger nail and sometimes others becoming black and blue and eventually beginning to detach from the nail bed. The bleeding of the nail bed and surrounding tissue results in the nail absorbing some of the blood and giving the characteristic bruised colour. This is, of course, quite painful and uncomfortable for the client and although a manicure could be performed on the rest of the hand, the affected nails should not be touched.

However, onycholysis is often a sympton of a systemic illness. Any illness which impairs the peripheral circulation could be the cause of this distressing nail condition, which tends to affect older women and can sometimes be seen in cases of chronic chilblains. It is often encountered in the feet. Once again this can be attributed to a knock or blow. In young women one often sees a shedding and bruised nail on the foot as a result of a sporting accident, such as a horse stepping on the foot. One such case was a client who constantly shed her large toenails due to the repeated trauma of her running shoes – she was a track athlete – rubbing against the nail. Eventually it was necessary for her to have running shoes custom made for her.

With care most cases of onycholysis will be cured when the damaged nail drops off and the new nail grows in its place. However, *with care* must be re-stated. The client must be warned that if anything damages the nail bed during the transitional period, the new nail may not form a proper attachment to the nail bed and any nail growing will be continuously shed. This condition would need medical treatment.

Paronychia

This is the next most frequently encountered condition. It is an inflamed condition of the soft tissue surrounding the nail and in advanced stages the nail bed. Usually caused by damage to the skin or by biting the cuticles, a bacterial infection then sets up and unless treated with great care can also damage the matrix area.

This is a definite contra-indication to manicure.

Hang nails (sometimes called agnails)

Often due to allowing the cuticle to be overgrown and dried, the cuticle splits and becomes uncomfortable.

If a bacterial infection sets up, then the condition becomes the former – paronychia. Great care should be taken with such infections as they do contra-indicate manicure.

Onychocryptosis

A long name for a common complaint, ingrowing nails. Usually found predominantly in the toenails, it can sometimes affect finger nails. Caused by a small spicule or sharp piece of nail being left behind during cutting or filing the nail. This spicule of nail then grows into the surrounding soft tissue causing it to become infected. Often granulation tissue builds up around it.

It can be avoided by not filing the nails too deeply in sulcus at the outer edges. It occurs more frequently in toe nails because they are usually more convoluted. This means that the nail has a very convex shape to it and the side edges of the toe nails tend to be more deeply buried in the sulcus of the nail bed. Great care should be taken when cutting the toe nails to ensure that the corners are neatly trimmed and no shards of nail remain. Many theories have been put forward over the years on how to avoid such a condition. The one that seems to continue is that of cutting a V in the centre of the nail. Research by eminent chiropodists has proved that this has no effect whatsoever on the condition, but does irritate the client due to tights and stockings becoming constantly caught on the V.

Onychocryptosis is a contra-indication to manicure or pedicure of the affected nail.

Onychorrhexis

This could almost be renamed the housewife's nails! A general term given to split or brittle nails. A few cases could be the result of a serious illness, but the majority are due to neglect. Anything which destroys the natural oils and moisture content of the nails and surrounding tissues could be the cause of this condition. Repeatedly immersing the hands in water with detergents or other strong chemicals without wearing gloves is the main offender. Also some occupations where certain chemicals are used could cause this. However, nowadays, this is not likely as most working conditions are closely monitored by safety officers and rubber gloves would be issued.

Ironically, it can also occur where a client does really take a great pride in her hands and is constantly manicuring them. Too much nail varnish remover, particularly one that contains acetone, over-zealous use of manicure equipment around the cuticles and the too-frequent use of excessive amounts of cuticle remover can also cause this condition. Great care should be taken by the manicurist when treating such nails and a good routine of home care should be established as soon as possible.

Onychophagy

Usually seen in young women of nervous attitudes, onychophagy is the medical name for nail biting. This occasionally only involves one nail, but in most cases the nails of both hands are involved. Sometimes these are bitten to such an extent that the cuticles and surrounding soft tissues are involved, often with a resulting infection and paronychia. Often this has a spontaneous cure when a romantic relationship develops, but on occasions the person continues to nail bite well into maturity.

Where a manicure can be done it should be done with great sympathy and the client should be encouraged to try to stop this terrible habit, which is usually very distressing to the client. There are many 'cures' on the market, usually harmless chemicals for painting on the nails which taste foul when bitten. Some clients may find success with one of these, but the majority find them ineffective.

Onychauxis (or hypertrophied nail)

This is an excessive overgrowth of nail, either in thickness or in length, usually the result of trauma or a serious illness. It is more often encountered on the nails of the feet, and can be quite unsightly if the client wishes to wear summer sandals. If an electric drill is not available, the client should be referred to her local State Registered Chiropodist who will drill it down for her.

Onychogryphosis
This is very similar to onychauxis except that the overgrowth of the nail manifests itself in a very thickened, ridged curvature of the nail, often called a 'rams horn nail' because of its likeness to a rams horn. Once again, nearly always encountered in the feet, although it can sometimes appear on the thumb nail of the hand. To attempt to cut or file it with ordinary manicuring equipment would be out of the question, so once again this should be referred to a State Registered Chiropodist.

Psoriasis
This very unpleasant but non-infectious skin condition produces large patches of reddened, dry skin which is usually covered in dry silvery scale-like patches of shedding skin. It is said to be of nervous origin but it usually affects women much more than men. One of its unpleasant symptoms is a chronic pitting of the nail. Usually only the finger nails are affected, but it causes great embarrassment and distress to sufferers. The pits are scattered irregularly over the nail plate. The pitting can be so severe in some cases that the nail bed is exposed and in some instances becomes infected. If this condition is not treated medically the nail will shed and may not grow again. Nails with this condition should never be manicured.

Tinea Pedis – ringworm of the feet – athletes foot
An infectious condition of the feet which is known by all the names above. Usually spread over the foot and between the toes, this unpleasant complaint is often found in women who do a lot of sport and wear rubber-soled shoes for hours at a time with the feet becoming rather hot. Also people in certain occupations tend to suffer from this; namely where they have to work in very moist warm conditions such as a bakery or an hotel kitchen. It is a very itchy condition with the vesicles breaking open in acute conditions and the whole area appearing red and oozing. This is of course a contra-indication to pedicure and is the first thing that should be looked for. When the fungal infection spreads to the nails it becomes:

Onychomycosis – Tinea Unguium – ringworm of the nail
Quite a common disease mainly of the toe nails, but can
sometimes be seen in the nails of the hands. There are several
types and generally they discolour the nail (it looks decidedly
unhealthy), some have pus in the nail sulcus, and the most serious
form destroys the layers of the nail itself. These layers then in turn
peel away to reveal further infected nail tissue below. It is a contra-
indication to manicure or pedicure.

Verruca Pedis
A very troublesome type of wart of the foot, which is very
contagious. The symptoms are usually a throbbing pain in one
area of the foot and the feeling of constantly walking on a sharp,
painful object. The warts are an accumulation of soft cells which
appear rather like a small sponge growing on the foot. This
condition is very much the concern of the State Registered
Chiropodist and should contra-indicate pedicure.

———

These are the most common nail, foot and hand conditions one
is likely to encounter. There are more, but they are unlikely to be
encountered in the normal salon practice. However the therapist
who is interested in furthering her knowledge of the subject
should read *Nails in Disease* by Peter D Samman.
A far more common reason for damaged and diseased nails
regrettably is manicuring and cosmetics. It cannot be stressed
strongly enough that a great many nails are damaged through
manicure instruments being used too roughly. Many nails are also
subject to allergies and it has been proved that many women are
allergic to nail varnish, base coats, nail varnish removers and most
of all cuticle removers.
Another cause for concern has been the number of women who
have reacted to nail hardeners, particularly those that contain
formaldehyde.
There is also a growing number of women now with nails and
nail beds severely damaged by the wearing of built-on nails. Many
are allergic to the chemical composition of some of the acrylic
type nails. Disastrously, their attempts to cover up damaged or
breaking nails have resulted in an even more unsightly case of
allergic reactions with not only the nail plate and bed becoming
involved, but also the cuticles and surrounding soft tissue.

This is, of course, most unfortunate as many thousands of women have been very pleased with the results of the build-on nails and have been wearing them for some years now with no ill effects.

The problem of allergic reactions is a very worrying one, and one finds that many clients who have become sensitised by one type of cosmetic tend to start reacting to almost everything. In instances of this kind, it is far better to dissuade the client from having treatment rather than run the risk of triggering off a new set of allergies for her.

Discoloration of nails

A frequently encountered problem is that of nail discoloration. One often sees instances of badly discoloured nails due to the use of certain dyes or chemicals used in working situations. Indeed therapists themselves can sometimes inadvertently badly stain their own nails by contaminating them with eyelash tint. Hairdressers are also vulnerable to tint stains, as are some clients involved in photographic development work.

The taking of certain strong drugs for a systemic illness can also cause a change in the colour of the nail bed.

However, the two main causes appear to be either smoking or the use of nail varnish. With the decrease in the number of women smoking one does not encounter quite so much now the heavily nicotine stained hands of a few years ago, in which the nails often appeared a dark orangey-yellow. This, in some instances, can be removed with an application of a nail whitener such as *Perox Chlor*.

By far the most common reason for badly stained and discoloured nails though is the practice of applying nail varnish containing the very dark red pigments directly on to the nail, without the use of a clear colourless base coat. The pigment 'bleeds' into the nail plate and usually does not lighten until the stained portion has grown up the nail and been filed away.

A good manicurist should instruct her client how to avoid such problems when she is doing her own manicure at home.

6 Materials and products

Study of materials and products used in manicure and pedicure

The study of the composition and preparation of the materials used in manicure and pedicure is a fascinating one. Those who have the facilities of a laboratory, as in most colleges today, can even try their hand at producing some of the creams and cosmetics themselves. Many of the ingredients are easily obtained, but with some of the more complicated ingredients, it would be necessary to order them from a specialist supplier. However, the simpler products could easily be made as a practical exercise. Those students who have had the benefit of recent chemistry classes may have already had the opportunity to make some of the standard products, as many sixth form chemistry classes use simple cosmetics as a class project.

Nail varnish removers
These are usually a simple mixture of acetone, glycerine and perfume. However, the problem is that acetone has a very strong drying action on the nail surface and also the surrounding tissue if allowed to flood the nail. Various manufacturers have attempted to counteract this by replacing the acetone with water miscible solvents such as ethyl acetate.

Another method of attempting to counteract the drying effect has been by blending the solvents together with lanolin and waxes to produce a cream nail enamel remover. Removers have a high evaporation rate, so that care should be taken to replace the cap as soon as it has been used. It should never be poured into an open container and left on the manicure table as it evaporates and it becomes a noxious vapour, particularly in a small enclosed cubicle. Large quantities of varnish remover should be stored in a cool dry place well away from direct sunlight or any form of heat.

Cuticle removers
Cuticle removers are normally an alkaline solution produced in either liquid or cream form. Original formulae were basically dilutions of varying strengths of potassium hydroxide. However, additives were needed because of the high evaporation rate and to counteract the risk of irritation of the skin. Humectants were added in the form of glycerine or propylene glycol.

Because of the extreme drying effect achieved by the use of cuticle removers it is suggested that they be used sparingly and washed off as soon as possible.

If manufacturing these on a project, it must be noted that the containers should be clearly labelled to the effect that a strong alkali is contained therein and the name of the alkali should be clearly stated.

Cuticle creams or softeners

Rich emollient creams form the basis of most of this type of product which is used for softening the cuticles. Sometimes quaternary ammonium compounds are used because of their affinity for protein. Lanolin and/or urea is often used in the attempt to soften the cuticle before mechanical removal.

Nail varnish or lacquer

Nail varnish or lacquers are one of the most popular items of modern cosmetics. Many women who do not wear any form of facial cosmetics at all will often wear nail varnish. The present highly sophisticated formulae have evolved over the years as fashion has changed from a very pale, shell pink and colourless varnish to the present strong dark colours which are the vogue today. The main essentials of a nail varnish is that it should be easy to apply, remain unchipped for as long as possible, have no adverse effect on the nail plate or surrounding soft tissue, and have a high degree of gloss finish.

The complicated formulae now contain film formers, such as nitro-cellulose; resins of the aryl-sulphonamide-formaldehyde type: plasticisers, solvents and colour pigments. The colour pigments used in nail varnishes must conform to the national legislation of their country of origin. This of course varies from country to country, but varnish manufactured in Britain must also conform to the EEC regulations on standards of purity and non-toxicity. Lists of permitted colours are issued by the appropriate authority.

Pearlised or irridescent lacquers are obtained by the inclusion of synthetic pearl pigments into the formula. The problem of irridescent lacquers has always been the tendency for the crystalline pigments to settle. This has been largely overcome by the introduction of the synthetic pigment, but this presents difficulties by adding to the viscosity of the lacquer causing problems of thickening. This is then counteracted by the addition of a dilutent such as alcohol or hydrocarbon. Where nail varnish or lacquer is purchased in large quantities for retail sale a strict rotation of stock control should be operated as stock may thicken and harden when left standing for long periods of time. It is much better, if possible, to buy in smaller quantities regardless of tempting bulk buying terms.

Nail varnish should always be stored in a cool place, away from direct sunlight or any form of artificial heat.

Hand cream and lotions

Most cosmetic creams are emulsions prepared by melting and blending different waxes, oils, water and other ingredients. The main requirement in a hand cream or lotion is that it should have a certain amount of oily protection for the skin of the hands, this is known as an emollient property. It should also be a humectant, which means it can obtain moisture from the atmosphere and retain it on the skin's surface. Other ingredients are added for varying reasons: preservatives to prevent the waxes and oils from becoming rancid and perfumes to mask the sometimes unpleasant smell of some of the other ingredients.

Therapists often develop a distinct preference for a particular brand of cream or lotion, which they feel to be more effective than others. This often leads to recommending its use to clients when they ask for advice on home care. It makes sound business practice to have retail sizes of these creams readily available for purchase. It should, however, be left to the client to decide if she wants to purchase. Nothing is more certain to lose the client if she feels that she cannot attend for treatment without being pressurised into buying other items.

Nail whiteners

There are two distinct types of nail whiteners. The pencil, which is moistened and then run under the free edge of the nail, leaves a powdery white deposit under the free edge, thus causing it to appear much whiter when viewed from the other side. This is not normally used if the client has chosen a heavily coloured varnish, and is more usually used when the nail is covered with a colourless lacquer, or when buffed only, as in male manicures. Nail whitening pencil formulae usually have as their main active ingredient either zinc oxide or titanium dioxide.

Nail bleaches are usually a cream or paste and are effective not only for whitening under the free edge, but also for removing stains such as nicotine or vegetable and fruit stains from the nail plate and surrounding skin. Most contain hydrogen peroxide. One of the most effective on the market is 'Perox Chlor' produced by Ernest Jackson & Co Ltd of Devon.

Nail strengtheners

To counteact the dry brittle flaking nails, it is necessary to use and recommend for home use a nail strengthener and hardener. Many have appeared in the past few years, some with very much greater effectiveness than others. The formulae of these products are as varied as the products themselves, but most of them contain formaldehyde in some form or other. However, formaldehyde is a known sensitiser and has been known to produce extensive problems to users.

Some nail varnish manufacturers now incorporate nail hardening additives in their varnishes in an attempt to overcome the problem. Other nail strengtheners are produced in the form of a colourless base coat type of varnish. The best of this type is undoubtedly *Nail Magic*, an American product which is marketed in the UK by Jica Ltd of Chertsey, Surrey. The active ingredient in this product is a powder which settles out when left standing.

Care should be taken to ensure that the powder is evenly distributed by thorough shaking before use and also the client should be instructed to do the same, as this treatment should be followed up faithfully by the client at home.

Massage cream

Creams suitable for massage should be non-absorbent so that the therapist's hands can slide over the skin of hands, arms, feet and legs without any 'drag', particularly where there is a lot of hair present. Care must also be taken to select a non-irritant or hypo-allergenic cream.

The busy manicure and pedicure cubicle is not the place to be doing time-consuming patch testing. Besides which, the modern client has neither the time nor inclination for such procedures: she expects her therapist to be conversant with all the latest products and this definitely includes creams that are proven non-irritant.

A very good example of this type of cream is the *Queen Cosmetics* massage cream. This contains in its formula liquid paraffin, paraffin wax, beeswax, petrolatum, and p-hydroxybenzoates. This cream has solid cream consistency whilst in the jar, but melts to an oily consistency on contact with the skin, making it an ideal product for massage. It can easily be removed at the completion of the massage routine by either surgical spirit or the more pleasant to use eau de Cologne.

Suppliers of equipment and materials

The manicure and pedicure equipment and materials mentioned in this book can be obtained from the following suppliers:

Aston and Finchers
Cash & Carry Wholesalers, 8 Holyhead Road, Birmingham B21 OLY
And their ten other branches at: Birmingham, Bristol, Cardiff, Swansea, Plymouth, Coventry, Nottingham, and Liverpool

Ellisons
Cash & Carry and Mail Order wholesalers, Brindley Road South, Exhall, Coventry

Mavala International Ltd
Leroy House, 436 Essex Road, London N1

The Scholl Manufacturing Co
Scholl UK Ltd, 182–204 John Street, London EC1P

Hypo-allergenic hand cream and massage cream:
Queen Cosmetics Ltd, 130 Wigmore Street, London EC1

Solar Nail Products
Fabricius Martin, 45 Highlands Heath, Portsmouth Road, London SW15

Training establishments

Specialising in teaching manicure and pedicure techniques and allied subjects.

The Mavala Manicure School
139a New Bond Street, London W1Y 9FB

Fabricius Martin (Solar Nails)
45 Highlands Heath, Portsmouth Road, London SW15 3TX

Internation Health and Beauty Council
24 River Road, Arundel, West Sussex BN18 9EY

British Association of Beauty Therapy and Cosmetology
   (Secretariat)
Suite 5, Wolseley House, Oriel Road, Cheltenham, Glos

Index